JOB DESCRIPTIONS
TRAINING SCHEDULES
FOR THE VETERINARY TEAM

Growing Your Business Knowledge

Welcome to the world of veterinary law and practice management. The Banc of America Practice Solutions™ group is pleased to team up with Dr. James Wilson and Priority Press, Ltd. to make this book available to VBMA officers and members. We trust that it will help stimulate and prepare you for the ownership of a veterinary practice someday. We realize that as you study hard to learn the basic and clinical sciences, that goal may not be your top priority.

Our hope is that by stimulating your interest in business while you are a student, you will be ready to accept the challenge of practice ownership within a reasonable time after graduation. Please accept that when money is needed to start or buy a veterinary practice, our team will be there to help.* For materials that we can provide to help in the process, including while you area a student, please be sure to contact one of us for assistance.

Best of luck completing the requirements needed to become a *real doctor*, i.e., a one that treats more than a single species.

Ian Widensky, VP Banc of America Practice Solutions
ian.widensky@bankofamerica.com

888-600-9612

*All programs subject to credit approval and loan amounts are subject to creditworthiness. Some restrictions may apply. Banc of America Practice Solutions™, Inc. is a subsidiary of Bank of America Corporation. Banc of America Practice Solutions™ and Bank of America are registered trademarks of Bank of America Corporation.

Job Descriptions and Training Schedules for the Veterinary Team

James F. Wilson, DVM, JD and
Karen Gendron, DVM

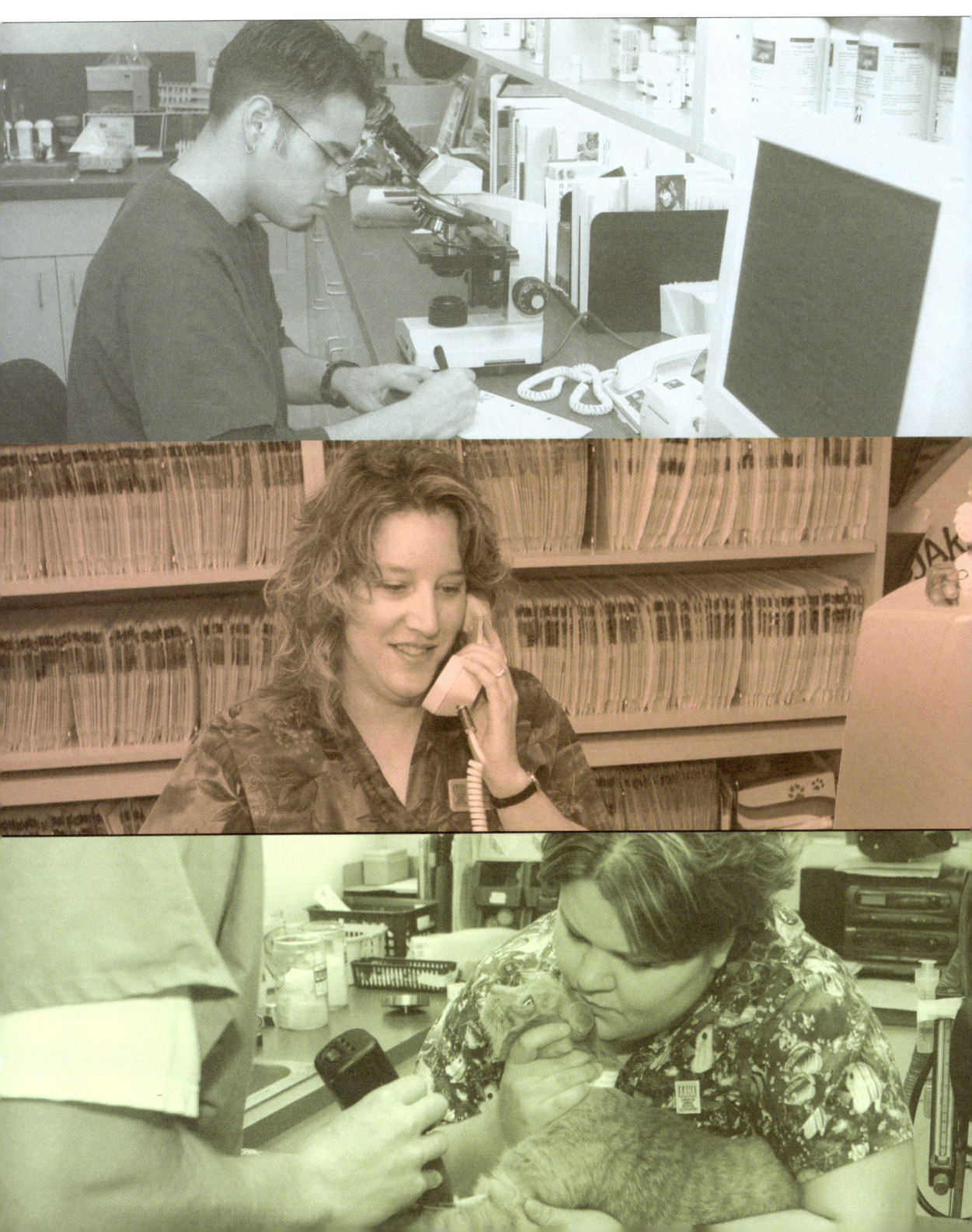

Managing Editor: Elise P. Wilson
Production: Sheridan Books, Inc., Ann Arbor, MI

James F. Wilson, DVM, JD
  Adjunct Associate Professor, University of Pennsylvania School of Veterinary Medicine; Visiting Lecturer, Colorado and North Carolina State University Schools of Veterinary Medicine; Proprietor, Priority Veterinary Management Consultants, Yardley, PA

Karen Gendron, DVM

© 2005 by Priority Press, Ltd.
Second Printing 2009
All rights reserved

Reproduction or translation of any part of this work beyond that permitted by Section 107 or 108 of the 1976 United States Copyright Act without the permission of the copyright owner is unlawful. Requests for permission or further information should be addressed to: Permissions Department, Priority Press, Ltd., 2111 Yardley Rd., Yardley, PA 19067.

Library of Congress Cataloging in Publication Date:

Wilson, James, 1943-
  Job Descriptions and Training Schedules for the Veterinary Team

ISBN 0-9621007-4-9

Printed in the United States of America

10 9 8 7 6 5 4

TABLE OF CONTENTS

Dedication	xiii
Acknowledgments	xv
Preface	xvii

Chapter 1 • Basics of Job Descriptions

Why Job Descriptions Are Important	1
Organizational Reasons	1
Educational Reasons	2
Legal Reasons	2
Job Descriptions as Management Tools	7
Employee Recruitment	7
Applicant Selection	8
Employee Training	8
Employee Evaluations	9
Employee Compensation	9
Making Job Descriptions SMART	11
Specific	11
Measurable	11
Achievable	12
Relevant	12
Time-Sensitive	12
Customizing Job Descriptions	13
Training Schedules	15
Customizing Training Schedules	16

Chapter 2 • Receptionist Job Description

General Knowledge and Tasks	19
General Knowledge	19
General Tasks	20
Client-Interaction Tasks	20
Face-to-Face Client-Interaction Tasks	21
Client-Interaction Telephone Tasks	23
Doctor/Technician-Support Tasks	23

General Telephone Tasks	24
Medical-Record Management Tasks	25
Daily Medical-Record Preparation Tasks	25
Medical-Record Filing Tasks	25
General Medical-Record Tasks	25
Reception-Area and Front-Office Tasks	26
Front-Office Management Tasks	26
Reception-Area Housekeeping Tasks	26
Supplies-Management Tasks	27
Other Reception-Area Tasks	27
Computer Tasks	28
General Computer Tasks	28
Database-Management Tasks	29
Word-Processing Tasks	29
Report-Generation Tasks	29
Internet-Based Tasks	30
Financial Tasks	30
Cash-Management Tasks	30
Daily Closing Financial Tasks	30
Payment-Processing Tasks	30
Tasks Related to Incomplete Payments	31

CHAPTER 3 • RECEPTIONIST TRAINING SCHEDULE

Week One	33
Month One	35
Month Three	39
Month Six	41

CHAPTER 4 • VETERINARY ASSISTANT JOB DESCRIPTION

General Knowledge and Tasks	45
General Knowledge	45
General Tasks	46

Contents

Front-Office Tasks	47
Client-Interaction Tasks	48
Patient-Admittance Tasks	48
Pet-Identification Tasks	49
Patient-Discharge Tasks	49
Medical-Record Management Tasks	50
Exam-Room Tasks	51
Nursing-Care Tasks	52
Basic Patient-Care Tasks	52
Patient-Treatment Tasks	53
Technical Tasks	54
General Technical Tasks	54
Emergency-Care Tasks	55
Surgical-Assistance Tasks	55
Surgical Cleaning Tasks	56
Radiology Tasks	56

Chapter 5 • Veterinary Assistant Training Schedule

Week One	57
Month One	58
Month Three	62
Month Six	64

Chapter 6 • Veterinary Technician Job Description

General Knowledge and Tasks	67
General Knowledge	67
General Tasks	68
Front-Office Tasks	69
Client-Interaction Tasks	69
Patient-Admittance Tasks	69

Pet-Identification Tasks	70
Procedural Tasks	70
Patient-Discharge Tasks	70
Medical-Record Management Tasks	71
Exam-Room Tasks	72
Nursing-Care Tasks	73
Basic and Environmental Tasks	73
Patient-Treatment Tasks	73
Technical Tasks	75
General Technical Tasks	75
Emergency-Care Tasks	75
Laboratory Tasks	76
Surgical Tasks	77
Surgical Cleaning Tasks	78
Dental Tasks	78
Anesthetic Tasks	79
Imaging Tasks	80
Radiology Tasks	80
Ultrasound and Endoscopy Tasks	81
Inventory-Management Tasks	81

CHAPTER 7 • VETERINARY TECHNICIAN TRAINING SCHEDULE

Week One	92
Month One	94
Month Three	96
Month Six	96
Month Twelve	98

CHAPTER 8 • KENNEL ASSISTANT JOB DESCRIPTION

General Knowledge and Tasks	99
General Knowledge	99
General Tasks	99
Client-Interaction Tasks	101
Patient-Admittance Tasks	101

Patient-Discharge Tasks	102
Pet-Care Tasks	102
Examination and Restraint Tasks	102
Contagious-Disease Tasks	103
Pet-Care and Monitoring Tasks	103
Grooming Tasks	105
Kennel Procedures and Maintenance Tasks	105
Patient-Transfer and Record-Keeping Tasks	105
Cage-Cleaning Tasks	106
Facility-Maintenance Tasks	106

Chapter 9 • Kennel Assistant Training Schedule

Week One	107
Month One	109
Month Three	112
Month Six	113

Chapter 10 • Kennel Manager Job Description

General Knowledge and Tasks	115
General Knowledge	115
General Tasks	116
Client-Interaction Tasks	117
Patient-Admittance Tasks	117
Patient-Discharge Tasks	118
Pet-Care Tasks	119
Examination and Restraint Tasks	119
Pet-Care and Grooming Tasks	119
Kennel Procedures and Maintenance Tasks	121
Cage-Cleaning Tasks	122
Facility-Maintenance Tasks	122
Managerial Tasks	123
General Managerial Tasks	123
Hiring Tasks	124
Training Tasks	124
Performance-Appraisal and Termination Tasks	125

Chapter 11 • Office Manager Job Description

General Knowledge and Tasks	127
General Knowledge	127
General Tasks	127
Client-Interaction Tasks	128
Office Management Tasks	129
General Office-Management Tasks	130
Front-Desk Tasks	131
Phone Tasks	131
Computer and Internet Tasks	131
Forms, Handouts, and Medical-Records Tasks	132
Human-Resource Management Tasks	133
General Human-Resource Tasks	133
Hiring Tasks	134
Training Tasks	134
Performance-Appraisal and Termination Tasks	135
Pay and Benefit Tasks	135
Facility and Equipment Tasks	136
Financial-Management Tasks	137
Inventory-Management Tasks	139
Marketing Tasks	140

Chapter 12 • Practice Manager/Hospital Administrator Job Description

General Knowledge and Tasks	141
General Knowledge	141
General Tasks	141
Client-Interaction Tasks	142
Office-Management Tasks	143
General Office-Management Tasks	143
Phone Tasks	144
Computer and Internet Tasks	144
Procedure and Policy Tasks	145
Regulatory Tasks	146

Human-Resource Management Tasks	146
General Human-Resource Tasks	146
Hiring Tasks	147
Performance-Appraisal and Termination Tasks	148
Pay and Benefits Tasks	149
Facility and Equipment Tasks	149
Financial-Management Tasks	150
Inventory-Management Tasks	152
Marketing Tasks	153

Resources   155

DEDICATION

Dedicated to the support staff, clients, and my former partners, Drs. Bob Luebke, Laura Becker, and Joan Shaeffler, at Four Corners Veterinary Hospital in Concord, California, where I learned much of what appears in this book.

—Jim Wilson, DVM, JD

Dedicated to my family for sharing their love, support, and wisdom during all my endeavors.

—Karen Gendron, DVM

ACKNOWLEDGMENTS

Thanks to Elise Wilson, who has edited dozens of journal articles, five books, and hundreds of other documents for Jim. She greatly improved each and every one of them. Thanks also to Steve Kellner, whose office administration talents for Priority Veterinary Consultants freed up enough time to allow for the birth of this book.

Thanks to Vladimar Burkanov, the Russian-American scientist who invited Jim to serve as the veterinary anesthetist for Steller sea lions on an anesthesia and branding trip to the Kurile Islands in Russia during the summer of 2003. And to Elise for encouraging Jim to go on this once-in-a-lifetime scientific excursion, during which he could use his free time to compile nearly half of the original material contained herein. Moreover, it was Vladimar's satellite phone link that allowed for routine communication with Karen Gendron as we worked on many of the job descriptions and training schedules contained herein.

Last, and perhaps most important, thanks are in order to Erin Landeck at AAHA Press, who believed in the value of this project from its inception and coordinated everything to make it a reality. Without Erin's encouragement, this book would still be a dream waiting to come true.

PREFACE

Though it is an essential personnel-management task, practice managers and owners often forego defining what they expect of employees. Hiring new people without listing and explaining the tasks they are expected to complete leads to poor hiring decisions, disenchanted managers, and unhappy staff members. All too frequently, it also leads to rapid and costly staff turnover. It is equally troublesome not to provide existing staff members with clear expectations and measures of success that carve a path to merit raises and promotions.

Publications with brief veterinary-practice-specific job descriptions have been on the market for several years, but they offer minimal guidance for the immense volume of tasks associated with work in companion-animal practices. To prevent veterinary practices from being forced to invent and reinvent job descriptions, we have taken on this task with zeal. Our hope is that you can use these, customize them, and improve them to fit your needs and, in doing so, enhance the productivity and happiness of your entire staff—to your benefit and that of your clients, staff, and patients.

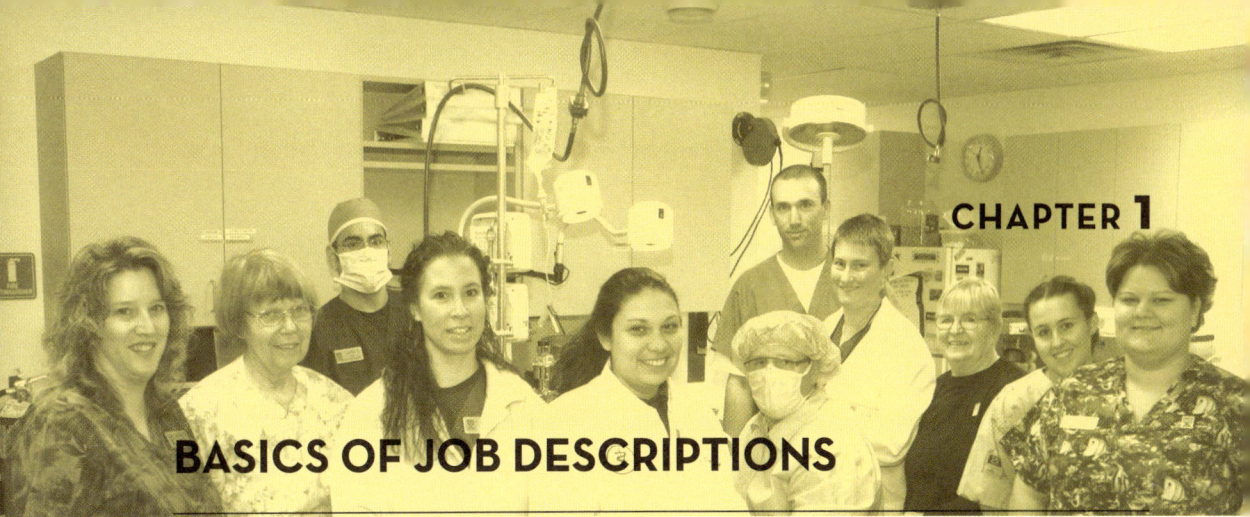

CHAPTER 1

BASICS OF JOB DESCRIPTIONS

Job descriptions are important organizational, educational, and legal tools for veterinary practices. Their primary purpose is to identify the essential functions and tasks associated with each position. The process of writing job descriptions forces the practice manager to clearly define what the job entails, and managers and applicants alike are able to immediately judge if the applicants are a good fit.

The secondary purpose of job descriptions is to clarify your expectations of existing employees and to paint a picture of the practice's organizational structure. A tertiary role of job descriptions is to provide a basis for training and evaluation.

Why Job Descriptions Are Important

Organizational Reasons

Personalized, thorough job descriptions set forth your medical and management philosophies as well as the practice's competencies. By describing in depth the responsibilities of each position, they communicate how each person can support the practice's mission and vision. Job descriptions also articulate how you assign work tasks.

For instance, technicians who are responsible for reporting mechanical problems with equipment can look to their job descriptions to find the chain of command. When receptionists are assigned the job of and given the authority to educate and assuage clients, they learn from the job description how you handle client relations. When the job description for kennel assistants indicates that cages or runs with urine or feces must be cleaned immediately, they understand your standards for cleanliness and patient comfort.

Educational Reasons

The precise wording found in the descriptions in this publication assists managers by identifying the manner in which tasks should be handled. For example, clients should not just be "greeted," they should be "greeted in a friendly and professional manner." Pets should not simply "be restrained," they should "be restrained in a manner that minimizes stress to them and the veterinary staff, while ensuring the safety of pets and people." Carefully worded tasks educate employees and provide the foundation for employee training schedules.

Prospective and existing employees also learn about the practice's equipment and capabilities by reading job descriptions. For example, if technicians are tasked with exposing and processing dental radiographs, they know that the practice provides that service. If assistants are expected to restrain birds, ferrets, pocket pets, and reptiles, they know the practice does not limit care to dogs and cats. When job descriptions include tasks for after-hours emergencies, new hires know the practice accepts emergencies and does not refer them. In this manner, job descriptions build a picture of the practice's equipment, services, and facility.

Legal Reasons

When applicants are assessed according to their abilities to perform the tasks set forth in the job descriptions, those who can best complete the tasks are more likely to be hired and promoted. If staff members question decisions about hiring or firing, job descriptions serve as references to evaluate whether employees were properly informed of and judged on their ability or inability to adequately perform the specified tasks. When any form of disciplinary action, demotion, or termination occurs, the job descriptions support the rationale for such decisions. For example, employees might be disciplined for failing to maintain client records in the manner outlined in their job descriptions or for failing to complete time cards as directed.

When measured against the job description, unsuccessful applicants or employees with negative performance appraisals and disciplinary actions will have great trouble convincing judges or arbitrators that they were not hired, denied advancement, or disciplined as a result of discriminatory decisions. Similarly, when lists of employees' accomplishments derived from detailed job descriptions are compared from one staff member to another, managers are able to legally defend their decisions for promotions or raises based on objective, nondiscriminatory assessments.

Understanding the Legal Impact of the ADA

We included specific physical abilities in these job descriptions in order to identify job tasks and support nondiscriminatory personnel policies in accordance with the Americans with Disabilities Act (ADA). Practices with 15 or more part-time and full-time employees who work twenty weeks or more per year must follow the standards set forth in the ADA. Specifically, this act prohibits discriminating against qualified applicants who have disabilities, as long as the disability does not prevent the employee from fulfilling the essential functions of the job. Essential job functions are those that employees must accomplish unaided or with reasonable accommodation. See the Resources section at the end of this book for excellent reference materials on this topic.

Identifying Essential Functions

Case law that interprets the Americans with Disabilities Act confirms that employers who have job descriptions help employees and themselves. This is particularly true when employers include descriptions of what are termed "essential job functions." This term means that the job duties to be performed are fundamental to the job rather than of marginal importance.

Employers use their own judgment as to what is essential, although their opinions are not always presumed to be correct. In other words, applicants who feel they suffered from discrimination can always challenge such assumptions. They would, however, face the legal difficulties inherent in overcoming such presumptions. When creating task lists, employers are not required to eliminate or transfer essential functions, i.e., fundamentally alter the nature of the job, in order to accommodate an employee with a disability.

In making determinations as to what functions are essential, employers should consider:

- whether or not a specific function must be performed by the person who fills that position;
- whether the function is already part of an existing job at that place of business;

- whether the responsibility for performing the function has been shared with others previously or is uniquely a part of the specific job for which this applicant is applying;
- whether written job descriptions were prepared before the job was advertised or applicants were interviewed, rather than after someone was hired;
- whether the terms of a collective bargaining agreement existed and were related to the function (rare in veterinary medicine);
- the amount of time spent performing the essential function relative to the total amount of time worked;
- what would happen to staff members who are currently (or who were formerly) in the position if they were (or had been) unable to perform the function;
- whether special training, a certain level or type of education, or a license is required;
- whether people performing similar work for other businesses perform this function;
- whether removing an essential function from the job fundamentally changes it; and/or what work is performed by incumbent staff members who do this job.

These considerations should be made with regard to each function of the job. No one factor is determinative; rather, all are considered together.

Suggested Formats for Job Descriptions

To best fulfill the requirements of the ADA, job descriptions should include the following ingredients:

A job title. Also include a department, if applicable.

A job purpose. This is a short summary of what the jobholder does. For example, a janitor may "complete general janitorial duties according to specifications."

Employee qualifications. These are important factors to consider when screening job applicants. The ADA does not restrict an employer's ability to establish education-related requirements, such as "high school graduate" or "having completed an AVMA-accredited veterinary technician program," provided that such requirement is job related, consistent with the needs of the business, and not intended to screen out persons with disabilities.

Quantity or production standards. In a veterinary practice, production standards could be number of clients to be seen per day, number of dental cleaning procedures to be completed per month, or level of revenue to be generated per month.

Environmental conditions. Because of the possibility of allergies and exposure to zoonotic diseases, it is important to include environmental conditions in job descriptions for veterinary practices. Environmental conditions could be of special importance in ambulatory large-animal practices where weather-related concerns would be much more common than in small-animal veterinary practices. Employers may think this is obvious from the stated job name and purpose, but it is better to explain the situation explicitly than to assume it is understood.

Personal protective equipment. Listing necessary personal protective equipment and devices (e.g., wearing safety goggles and masks when performing dental prophylaxes or steel-toed boots while working in an ambulatory equine practice) could be important because some individuals with disabilities may be unable to wear such items.

Job tasks. These are the heart of the job description, including the identification of concrete ways in which employees are required to perform job tasks. For each task, employers should also identify the following four characteristics:

- Equipment, weights, and/or measures involved in the task
- The physical demands—There are physical requirements related to just about every job, including clerical, management, or professional positions. However, the physical demands for a receptionist will usually be considerably less taxing than those of a veterinary technician, assistant, or kennel worker.
- Frequency—For full ADA compliance, it is useful for employers to consider and accurately state the frequency of each job task that must be performed.
- Essential functions—As discussed previously, it is important to determine which job tasks constitute "essential functions" of the job.

The job descriptions in this book note when employees must handle fractious animals, which exposes employees to potential physical injury, and when there may be exposure to zoonotic diseases. Also, the job descriptions define tasks that entail heavy lifting, squirming animals, frequent bending, or long hours spent standing during shifts. And, because of potential exposure to a multitude of allergens, diseases, and animal sizes, temperaments, and behaviors, it is important that job descriptions delineate which species of animals or other workplace allergens or health risks that an employee may be exposed to.

Disabilities and Interviewing

During the course of interviewing and selecting employees, employers may ask all applicants to explain or demonstrate how, with or without reasonable accommodations, they will be able to perform essential job functions. The following questions are examples of permissible questions that you can ask because they are not likely to elicit information about a disability.

- After having read the job description, can you perform the functions of this job with or without reasonable accommodation?
- Please describe and demonstrate how you would perform the essential functions of this job.
- Can you meet the attendance and punctuality requirements of this job?
- Do you use any illegal drugs?
- Do you have the required certification, registration, or license required by the state to perform this job?

The questions that follow are examples of impermissible disability-related inquiries that are likely to elicit information about a disability:

- Do you have any disability?
- Do you have a disability that would interfere with your ability to perform this job?
- How many days were you sick last year?
- Have you ever filed a worker's compensation claim?
- What prescription drugs are you currently taking?

An employer may determine not to hire individuals with disabilities for job-related reasons if the employer cannot provide reasonable accommodation without undue hardship on the employer. If there are more qualified applicants without disabilities, employers are free to hire them. Keep in mind that the ADA is not an affirmative-action law. If the most qualified person for the job has a disability, though, you should not base a hiring decision on the applicant's need for an accommodation or questions regarding the applicant's performance of "marginal" functions. Your decision must focus on the ability of the applicant to perform the essential functions of the job.

In summary, Title I of the ADA does allow some discrimination. In doing so, it states that certain employers may discriminate against individuals with disabilities by not making reasonable accommodation for applicants or employees with known physical and mental limitations (or otherwise qualified individuals with disabilities) if they can show that the accommodation would impose an undue hardship on the operation of the business.

Job Descriptions as Management Tools

The job descriptions in this manual go well beyond a simplistic list of the essential tasks of each position. Consequently, they can be used effectively as management tools for employee recruitment, selection, training, evaluation, compensation, and promotion.

Employee Recruitment

When used properly, well-delineated and well-written job descriptions help managers draft more effective employment advertisements. And, good ads stimulate potential applicants to carefully assess their interest in and qualifications for that particular position. A classified ad written like this one fails to accomplish this mission:

> Receptionist needed. F/T position including some Saturdays. Send resume to Ms. Jane Doe, Office Manager, XYZ Veterinary Hospital, 123 Main Street, Anytown, PA 19067. 215/555-0000.

This ad is not likely to capture the attention of potential applicants or inform them of employers' expectations. Consider instead the following ad, which includes the key components of a job description:

> Veterinary practice seeks mature, friendly, efficient receptionist with strong phone/customer relations skills who appreciates the human-animal bond and likes pets and people. Accuracy and attention to detail critical. 35 hrs/wk, occ'l eves and Saturdays. Send resume to Ms. Jane Doe, Office Manager, XYZ Veterinary Hospital, 123 Main Street, Anytown, PA 19067. 215/555-0000.

Applicant Selection

Preceding the scheduling of a job interview, applicants should be required to read the job description for the position for which they are applying. During the interview itself, job descriptions should be used to trigger questions about the abilities, skills, and personalities of the applicants to ensure that they match the requirements of the position. More specifically, the job descriptions should serve as prehire checklists for technical and management positions.

Job descriptions allow managers to better assess which applicants best meet the requirements of the job. In addition, they help managers evaluate how much technical training will be required once an applicant is hired.

Employee Training

We have grouped the tasks for each job description to make them more understandable and less overwhelming. For example, trainers and managers can point out that, "The tasks in this group are all related to 'general telephone tasks.' Although there are many details here, we expect you to learn the ones in this group during your first week on the job." With that in mind, you can easily assign priority levels to groups of tasks within the training schedule, further customizing this process to fit your practice.

We have provided suggested training schedules for receptionists, technician assistants, technicians, and kennel attendants. These training schedules, which you can modify for each position and/or each employee, give new employees a clear timeline as to when they must be able to perform each task. For example, by the end of the first week, a kennel assistant should have learned to break down cages, including removing bedding to be washed, emptying and disinfecting food and water containers, and cleaning and disinfecting the cages. A receptionist should have learned, within the first month of employment, to answer questions about pricing in a manner that encourages potential clients to visit the practice.

Effective training requires knowledgeable and committed trainers, defined tasks to teach, and realistic time frames for newly hired staff to achieve proficiency. One or more trainers can be selected to teach each group of tasks. For example, a receptionist or office manager may teach a veterinary assistant about client relations and front-office tasks, while a technician will teach the assistant about exam-room and technical procedures. Once you assign trainers or mentors, you can work with them to ensure that they teach the new employee the required skills within the established time frame.

Employee Evaluations

When writing an employee's performance appraisal, evaluate how well the employee performed specific tasks listed in the job description for that position. You may select tasks that highlight each area of responsibility or only those that reflect a particular focus. For example, if you want to emphasize the development of the staff member's computer skills, you might evaluate many or all tasks from the computer skills list in a particular job description.

A new emphasis on dentistry might mean a shift in the evaluation to concentrate on related tasks. For example, you could evaluate a receptionist's skill at promoting this service or a technician's ability to explain the medical value of the procedure to clients.

When developing and conducting performance evaluations for newly hired staff, you can set goals for the future based on tasks for which the staff has not yet been trained or those they have failed to master. These tasks, in the form of an updated training-schedule checklist, can serve as the basis for setting goals and evaluating performance in subsequent evaluations. You can also use the training schedules to show what training would be required for an employee to be promoted to the next grade or level.

Evaluating employees' performance against their job descriptions is also the primary step leading to demotions, disciplinary action, and/or termination.

Employee Compensation

Many of the tasks we've outlined in each job description have different levels of achievement. There is a difference in competency and value between employees with basic computer skills and those with advanced skills; between those who can merely assist with radiographs and those who can independently perform an upper- or lower-GI barium series. Employees who are able to perform a large number of technical tasks completely and efficiently are more valuable and deserving of higher compensation than those who cannot.

Many practices elect to break their job descriptions into different task sets for entry-level, midlevel, and highly skilled employees. Employees rated at higher levels must be proficient at all of the tasks required of lower-level employees as well as at additional, more challenging tasks. Employees at different competency levels are then assigned different pay scales.

Only highly skilled technicians, for example, can induce anesthesia, intubate patients, recognize and record ECG abnormalities, properly adjust radiograph settings to correct for prior faulty exposures, and/or perform ultrasound recordings. These skills clearly add value to the practice, and staff capable of performing these advanced tasks merit wages reflective of them. In the same vein, receptionists who are capable of successfully resolving complaints made by difficult clients merit higher wages than those who cannot.

Some practices use the mastery of new tasks as their principal method of determining eligibility for pay increases. Employees are given lists of tasks from the job description and are advised that learning certain skills precipitates specific and immediate pay raises. Assistants who have learned to set up rooms for ocular exams, accurately perform and evaluate fecal samples for intestinal parasites, and perform basic cytology on ear swabs, for example, might be rewarded with modest hourly pay raises. In these cases, staff members continue to build their pay rates only by gaining additional technical skills.

It is critical, however, that employers value and reward more than just technical skills. Employees with these skills are most valuable when they also have many of emotional intelligence skills that Daniel Goleman writes about in his books *Emotional Intelligence* and *Working with Emotional Intelligence*. These include self-confidence, accurate self-assessment, self-control, adaptability, optimism, a commitment to the goals of the group, political awareness, strong communication skills, an ability to collaborate and cooperate, a strong customer-service orientation, and an ability to understand and empathize with others. The job descriptions in this manual are unique in that they are not merely skill-based, but also attitude-based. These attributes are critical in a customer-service industry such as veterinary medicine and should always be included when considering an employee's eligibility for pay raises.

Making Job Descriptions SMART

To maximize the benefits of the job descriptions in this manual, we have made them SMART. This acronym means that the job descriptions list *S*pecific, *M*easurable, *A*chievable, *R*elevant, and *T*ime-sensitive job duties. As you modify the existing job descriptions and create new ones, it is important to make them SMART.

Specific

To provide value and encourage employers and employees to refer to their job descriptions repeatedly, these task lists must articulate narrowly defined and clear expectations. Those that are too basic or vague leave employees guessing about your expectations or insisting that the tasks in question are not their responsibility. "Take pet from front desk to kennel," will not help kennel assistants learn or perform their jobs as effectively as, "Walk or carry pets to the appropriate wards. Apply identification bands. Settle pets comfortably in their assigned cages and runs. Provide fresh water, if permitted, and clean bedding. Mark cages and runs with pets' cage cards. Properly label and place or store personal items left behind by owners."

Measurable

Assigned tasks must be written in a manner that allows employees to determine whether they have completed their tasks and whether the quality and quantity of effort met their employer's expectations. For example, "Answer the phone by the third ring," provides a quantified expectation, as opposed to "Answer phone," which gives no direction. If you use the job descriptions in conjunction with the corresponding training schedules, you can assess the employee's achievement of tasks within the given time frames.

For existing employees, supervisors should complete unbiased evaluations that measure each staff member's performance against the job description. In well-managed practices, managers may create additional performance measurement devices in the form of client surveys and audits of computer or medical-record entries. When these methods are used, they reduce the likelihood of biases, errors, or misinterpretations by the supervisors who are evaluating employees' performance.

Achievable

The tasks set forth in this manual are achievable so that newly hired personnel can be as successful as possible. For example, asking a veterinary assistant to "Discuss administration or application of products and potential side effects with owners as instructed by doctors or technicians," is an achievable task. Asking a veterinary assistant to, "Learn the therapeutic uses of every drug dispensed from the practice," is probably not achievable. Achievable tasks accelerate the training process and reduce the need for retraining because employees can get it right the first time.

Relevant

To ensure relevance, job descriptions should be customized to fit each position and the expectations for individual employees at the inception of their employment. Subsequently, they should be reviewed and contemporized no less than annually, preferably in conjunction with routine performance appraisals.

For example, changes to the equipment, pharmaceuticals, or medical or surgical protocols or procedures usually necessitate changes in job descriptions. New computer systems with additional features may precipitate adding reports to the receptionists' task list and omitting others. The addition of an automated CBC machine would require adding tasks for technicians. For example: "Each morning, run appropriate controls on the automated CBC equipment as directed in the manufacturer's operating manual (attached by a cord to the back of the machine). Perform automated CBCs as outlined in the operations manual by 9:00 am each day or as requested by attending veterinarians." Routinely updating job descriptions keeps employees abreast of your expectations and offers the added benefit of protection from employment-related lawsuits.

Time-Sensitive

The tasks listed in job descriptions are time-sensitive when they are transcribed into training schedules and assimilated into performance appraisals. Training schedules provide timelines for the performance of specific tasks. To be deemed acceptable, the employee must be able to perform the tasks within a given number of weeks or months a set forth in the training schedule.

Customizing Job Descriptions

To be most effective, you must customize the job descriptions in this manual to fit the needs of your practice. Neither job applicants nor existing employees can understand what is expected of them if the tasks on their job descriptions are unclear, incomplete, or inaccurate. In addition, in discrimination and wrongful termination suits, judges and juries most readily find against employers that lack clear and detailed job descriptions. So, to get the maximum benefit from the investment you've made in this resource, you must tailor the job descriptions to your needs.

To customize these job descriptions, simply copy the file from the CD to your hard drive and open it in a word processing application. When revising electronic versions of documents, first save a file copy under a new name to protect the original document, then properly label the customized document. A good way to do this is to create an electronic folder on your computer's hard drive entitled "job descriptions." Under that, create subfolders for each of the positions such as receptionist (or the more contemporary term "customer service representative"), veterinary technician (also called veterinary nurse), veterinary assistant, and kennel worker. Next, establish folders under these titles with the names of the employees who work in that capacity.

We recommend using the "save as" function in your word processing software to enter the newest file name, followed by a space, followed by the current date. This same procedure can be used to update modified documents. For example, a veterinary assistant job description might be stored in a file entitled "c: //Employees/job descriptions/vet assistants/Sally Brown's JD 7-1-05." By managing job descriptions in this manner, you can preserve all the verbiage in the original document for use when writing new job descriptions. You can also update or recreate job descriptions for existing employees and save them with new dates without destroying the prior versions.

Once you have saved the document to your hard drive, follow these guidelines:

1. Delete tasks that are irrelevant to your practice. For example, in noncomputerized practices, all computer tasks should be removed. If veterinary assistants work only in exam rooms, remove all surgical tasks from their lists. If kennel assistants never have client contact, omit client-interaction tasks.

Alternatively, you can cross out irrelevant tasks on the hard copies of descriptions photocopied from this book.

2. With staff input, rework the task lists so that they reflect the realities and subcategories of jobs at your practice. For example, job descriptions for exam-room veterinary assistants are quite different than those for surgical, treatment-room, or ward assistants.

    The descriptions that we've written include all of the tasks that veterinary assistants might be expected to complete in highly leveraged practices whose owners and managers delegate to a great extent. If you do not assign this vast array of tasks to your assistants, adjust your job descriptions accordingly by deleting irrelevant tasks on electronic versions or crossing out tasks on hard copies.

    If you have several "levels" of a certain position, each successively lower level should have fewer tasks in the job description. For example, with respect to receptionists, level II receptionists should have shorter job descriptions than level III receptionists. You can do this by deleting all the tasks that you deem to be "level III" from the job description for level II receptionists.

3. After deleting irrelevant items as described above, make additions or amendments based on your employees, procedures, and positions. To maximize the usefulness and quality of these lists, have existing personnel review them and ask for corrections and additions. Staff members know their jobs the best.

    Additionally, when an employee with a favorable employment history leaves the practice, make sure that the employee reviews the job description and accepts, rejects, amends, or modifies task listings. This procedure ensures the best match of a job description to the actual job when the next person fills the position.

4. Add details specific to your practice. For example, "Generate monthly reminders" might be altered to read, "Send comprehensive physical examination and immunization reminders on the first day of each month. Send service and prescription refill reminders by the 15th day of each month."

    Similarly, you might alter, "Walk dogs in fenced exercise areas," to read, "Walk dogs only in the fenced area at the back of the practice." Your practice might also offer a unique service that is not included in these job descriptions. If that is the case, add the tasks related to that unique service.

5. Effective managers will make adjustments, or have their existing staff members do so, no less than annually to accommodate changes in individual job descriptions that result from increased cross-training, changes in procedures, or training that has advanced a staff member to a higher skill level. At that time you could refer to the original job description template to add previously deleted items or include tasks from other job descriptions.

TRAINING SCHEDULES

Because the job descriptions contained herein are so extensive, managers and newly hired staff could easily become overwhelmed or get bogged down trying to determine the order in which tasks need to be learned. Without careful or frequent oversight, you may find that employees are working hard to learn more advanced tasks before they have mastered the basics. This results in frustrated or angry managers and disheartened employees because they are out of sync with each other's desired or expected learning curves. The training schedules we have included in this manual will help you create orderly outlines of tasks that should be learned in the first week, the first month, the initial three months, and the first six months.

Note that the tasks listed in the training schedules do not match every task in the job descriptions. The rationale for excluding some tasks is that a number of them are based on inherent abilities and, as such, cannot be taught. For instance, all of the job descriptions herein require the ability to lift 50 pounds. Most applicants will already have this ability. If not, the applicant won't, in most cases, go through the physical training required to get to that point. So this job requirement and others like it are not listed in the training schedule. Other tasks are excluded from the training schedule when the advising of employees of the expectation alone provides sufficient training. Managers would not train employees to be at work on time, for example, but they would include this expectation in the job description.

Obviously, if opportunities arise for an employee to learn more advanced tasks, the employee should learn those skills sooner rather than later. However, a staff member can gain confidence more rapidly if a manager does not assign all of the tasks on the eight-page list in the first week. Moreover, if a new employee is feeling overwhelmed by demands from managers and coworkers, the training schedule reaffirms that the employee is on track and can be used as a basis for discussion with supervisors when necessary.

Customizing Training Schedules

The order of tasks in the training schedules reflects the authors' experience in many different practices. To be effective in your practice, though, *it must be customized to fit your needs and desires.*

When you first start using the training schedules, customize them for newly hired employees by deleting tasks that are not performed at your practice, just as you did with the job descriptions. As you hire new employees, give them copies of the training timelines for their positions. Together, you and the new hire should assess current proficiencies. Check off the tasks in which the employee is already proficient on the hard copy of the training schedule or highlight in color only the ones that need attention on the electronic copy and reprint it. The remaining tasks on the schedule should include only those in which the new staff member lacks proficiency, and, consequently, the ones for which the employee will require specific or additional training. (Note: Additional specific recommendations to customize the veterinary technician training schedule are provided in that section.)

Discuss the weekly and monthly timelines presented in the training schedules with the trainees. Identify the resources that newly hired personnel will use for acquiring the knowledge and/or training they lack. At this time, introduce the employee to your reference textbooks, customized staff training and/or procedures manual, and video- or DVD-training library. Also explain web- or computer-based learning programs or off-site programs you use to train your employees. (See the Resource section at the end of this manual for ideas.)

Inform employees as to how and when they are expected to access training material. Set up regular progress checks to ensure that employees remain on track. When the employee has mastered a skill, highlight it in a different color or delete it from the training schedule, which then can be reprinted to list only those tasks that have yet to be mastered.

Alternatively, you can cross out or check off the skills that have been mastered on a hard copy of the training schedule. In this manner, training schedules are periodically updated and managers are forced to keep the training process on track. Hard copies of the new job descriptions or training schedules should be provided to employees as this process unfolds.

You can also use training schedules to identify deficiencies in the performance of existing employees or to identify new learning opportunities that will enable staff members to move to higher grade levels. Motivated employees will reference their task lists, independent of their managers, to determine where they need to improve.

Well-written and properly used job descriptions benefit everyone. Employers win because they are more apt to recruit, select, hire, retain, and promote people who add value to their practices.

Employees win because they now know what is expected of them, and they can refer to written lists of tasks for instructions and direction. They can also use the job descriptions to understand how to advance their careers and increase their compensation.

Clients win because their appointments will progress more efficiently, they will receive more consistent service, and they will be treated as valued customers. And, best of all, patients win because they receive a higher and more consistent level of care from a well-trained staff of compassionate and competent people.

CHAPTER 2

RECEPTIONIST JOB DESCRIPTION

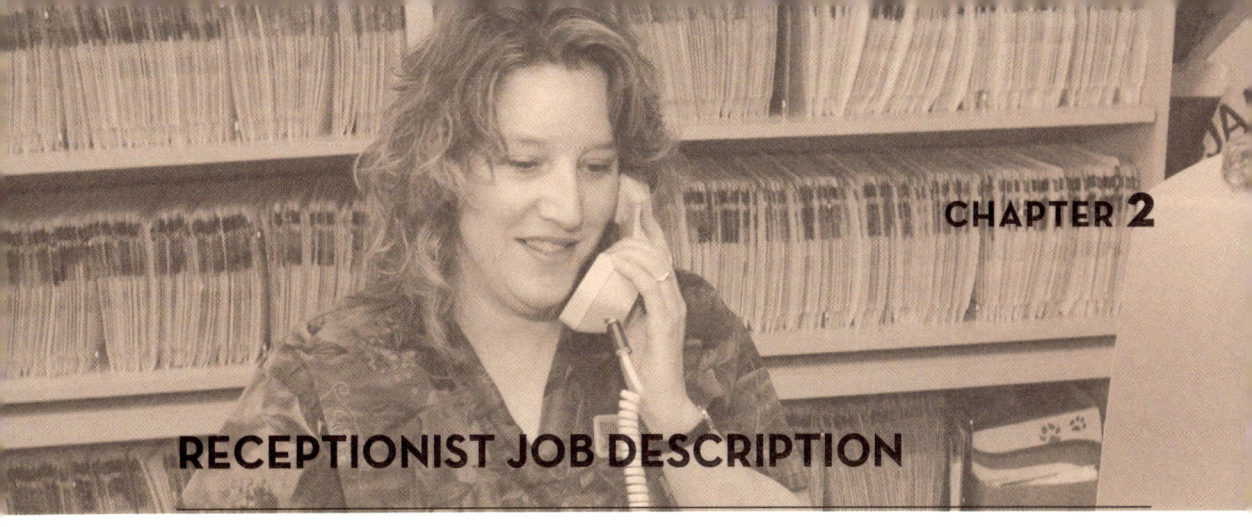

Receptionists (who are also called customer service representatives or client-relations specialists) are the customer-relations experts in a veterinary practice. They are the clients' first impression of the practice, on the phone or in person. Receptionists must possess strong organizational skills, excellent telephone and in-person communication skills, and the ability to remain calm under pressure. Receptionists must have compassion for animals and their owners and understand the stress that patients and clients endure.

Receptionists are responsible for greeting clients; differentiating routine cases from emergency cases; scheduling appointments; entering client, patient, and financial data into the computer; generating invoices and explaining them to clients; processing payments; and managing the retrieval and storage of medical records.

Receptionists should expect to spend nearly all of their workdays at the front desk. The position requires the completion of a high-school degree or further education, competence in the English language, patience, and a pleasant manner. Ideally, newly hired receptionists will possess computer skills and have had cashier and related front-office work experience.

General Knowledge and Tasks

General Knowledge

- Keep a street map readily retrievable, and give directions to the practice.
- Know the range of services the practice provides and the species it treats.
- Be reasonably familiar with breeds and coat colors.
- Follow OSHA standards. Be able to find Material Safety Data Sheets quickly.
- Know standard medical and business abbreviations.

- Use proper medical terminology when speaking and writing.
- Competently speak and write the English language.
- Competently speak a second language commonly used at the practice.
- Understand the life cycle and pathology of common parasites (intestinal parasites, heartworms, fleas, ticks), and know the names of most common preventatives, recommended treatments, and diagnostics.
- Be familiar with zoonotic (contagious) diseases, including their prevention and steps to reduce or eliminate transmission.
- Communicate with clients about the various pet-identification systems available, including tags, tattoos, and microchips.
- Know the policies regarding provision of veterinary care, treatment of stray animals, deposits for hospitalized patients, payments, credit, pet health insurance, and finance fees.

General Tasks

- Always be in position and prepared to work by the start of each scheduled shift.
- Maintain accurate personal time cards.
- Enter the practice through the front door so that you see what clients see. Routinely pick up trash or feces from the parking lot, sidewalks, or entryway.
- Maintain a professional appearance while at work, including clean and pressed uniforms or clothes. Change clothes daily as necessary to look professional and avoid carrying odors.
- Smile and maintain an even, friendly demeanor while on the job.
- Perform job tasks efficiently without rushing.
- Handle stress and pressure with poise and tact.
- Show respect for clients, team members, and animals (alive or deceased) at all times.
- Have the physical strength and ability to stand for an entire shift when needed, and be able to lift pets and objects weighing up to 50 pounds without assistance. Assist in lifting patients weighing more than 50 pounds.
- Prioritize tasks to maximize client satisfaction and patient health.

- Maintain a list of tasks and engage in productive work during slow periods.
- Assist other employees as needed. Take over for colleagues when they are called away to another priority.
- Read and refer to the personnel policy manual for answers to staff policy questions before asking the owner(s) or manager(s).
- Participate in your performance appraisal, and, as requested, in those of others.
- Participate in all staff and training meetings.
- Conduct tours of the practice and/or kennel. Before each tour, ensure that the facility is orderly and that staff and patients are prepared for tours.
- Maintain constant vigilance regarding open doorways that could allow pets to escape from the facility.
- Maintain strict confidentiality regarding clients and patients for whom the practice provides veterinary services.
- Be prepared to handle any facility emergency that may arise, including facility fire or weather-related emergencies. Follow contingency plans.
- Follow established closing procedures to ensure the security of patients, staff, data, revenue, inventory, and the facility.

Client-Interaction Tasks

Face-to-Face Client-Interaction Tasks

- Cordially greet arriving clients and patients, and address each by name.
- While handling phone calls, acknowledge the arrival of people in the reception area with eye contact and/or a hand wave.
- Review consent forms with clients and have clients sign the forms. Check that the clients' signatures match the signatures on the records.
- Advise clients of special call-in times to check on patients or speak with doctors.
- Using reminder, recall-system, and outpatient-visit and patient-admission protocols, advise clients of recommended services for their pets.

- Explain special programs offered by the practice.
- Advise clients of significant changes in policies or services since their last visit.
- Provide clients with accurate and thorough information about all over-the-counter products. Understand and explain internal- and external-parasite products as well as diets, dental products, and behavior management tools.
- Refer product questions you are unable to fully or accurately answer to doctors or technicians.
- Give estimates for services to be performed on patients.
- Provide clients with handouts and brochures regarding relevant medical conditions, surgeries, immunizations, internal and external parasites, pet insurance, and diets.
- Explain delays to clients. Ensure the comfort of clients and patients during their waits. Reschedule appointments as needed.
- Placate and/or compensate clients distressed by long waits, scheduling glitches, and other problems.
- Escort clients and patients to clean, empty exam rooms free of persistent, offensive odors.
- Assist clients with unruly or unrestrained pets. Ensure that all dogs are leashed and that cats and smaller pets are caged. Isolate aggressive pets. Request assistance as needed.
- Monitor patients' behaviors and note potentially aggressive behaviors. Use caution when handling aggressive or potentially aggressive pets. Request assistance when needed.
- Offer water to clients or patients in need (or withhold water from patients as appropriate).
- Handle angry or grieving clients in a calm, reassuring manner. Escort complaining or angry clients from the reception area to a separate, closed room where their complaints may be heard privately. When necessary, enlist a doctor or the office manager to resolve the complaint.
- Dispense prescribed medications and diets to clients. Discuss dosing and administration instructions to ensure that clients understand the use of prescribed products. Advise clients of common side effects of dispensed medications as instructed by doctors or technicians.
- Discharge hospitalized patients and boarded and groomed pets. Review discharge instructions and medications with clients. Give a copy of the instructions to the client and put a copy in the medical record. Discuss any problems noted in the record.

For hospitalized patients, schedule recheck (medical progress) appointments and follow-up callbacks.
- Provide basic grief counseling and arrange for more in-depth counseling for clients in need. Always be sensitive to background chatter or conversations that could exacerbate the anxieties and grief clients experience during euthanasias or deaths of their pets.
- Provide clients with information regarding options available for the remains of deceased pets.
- Assist clients to their cars if necessary.
- Distribute puppy, kitten, and new patient kits.

Client-Interaction Telephone Tasks
- Use clients' and patients' names during conversations.
- Schedule appointments for exams, rechecks, surgeries, medical procedures, boarding, and grooming.
- Call clients with hospitalized pets to provide patient status updates.
- Provide basic pricing information to callers. Respond in a manner that encourages potential clients to visit the practice.
- Answer routine questions or refer callers to the appropriate colleagues.
- Receive and record prescription-refill requests.
- Schedule euthanasias to maximize the comfort of clients and patients while allowing the practice to run efficiently.
- Schedule house calls according to written guidelines.
- Call clients scheduled for the next day to remind them of their appointments, appointment times, and special instructions, such as the need for fasting or withholding or administering medications.
- Call clients on the callback lists to check on patients' well-being and answer questions.
- Call clients who missed appointments and reschedule their appointments.

Doctor/Technician-Support Tasks
- Seek the assistance of doctors or technicians immediately when assessing potentially critical patients.

- Verify and obtain approval from a veterinarian prior to dispensing or delivering medication to a client.
- Ensure that doctors, technicians, and assistants enter occupied exam rooms within reasonable time periods.
- Obtain current patient-status reports or updates from doctors, technicians, or assistants.
- Prepare medications and prescriptions for dispensing as directed by the doctor. Ensure that each prescription label contains the following information: doctor's name; practice's name, address, and phone number including area code; date; patient's and client's name; medication name, strength and volume (or number); administration instructions including route of administration, such as by mouth or in the ear; and product's expiration date.
- Inform the practice manager or doctors immediately of all bite or scratch wounds you suffer so that reports can be made and you can be referred for timely medical care by a physician, if necessary. Clean all wounds quickly and thoroughly.

General Telephone Tasks

- Know phone functions, including hold, intercom, transfer, forward, and three-way calling.
- Answer the phone by the third ring and use the recommended greeting.
- Smile while answering and talking on the phone to enhance the friendly quality of your voice.
- Manage multiple phone lines effectively; prioritize phone calls.
- Follow the written telephone scripts.
- Transfer calls to the answering service or set the answering machine to accept calls during staff meetings and hours during which the practice is closed. Stop transfer of calls to the answering service or turn off the answering machine when staff members are available to receive calls.
- Call in prescriptions to outside pharmacies.
- Transcribe messages from the answering machine and distribute messages appropriately.
- Accurately record messages for doctors and staff. Note the caller's name, date, time of call, return phone number, and message. Notify recipients of urgent messages immediately. Place routine messages in the appropriate communication boxes.

Medical-Record Management Tasks

Daily Medical-Record Preparation Tasks
- Pull charts for incoming clients.
- Upon the client's arrival, mark the patient's medical record with the date and a brief synopsis of the reasons for the visit.
- Check for and enter phone, address, and email updates in clients' records.
- Check for and enter medical updates (spay/neuter status, immunization status, microchip number) in patients' medical records.
- Attach a travel or circle sheet marked with the patient's and client's names to the medical record of each arriving client.
- For patients that are being admitted, attach cage cards and completed client-consent or other forms to the medical record.

Medical-Record Filing Tasks
- Understand the medical-record filing system.
- Know all possible locations for storage of records of hospitalized patients.
- Properly use bins or slots assigned to doctors, staff, pharmacy, lab, and callbacks.
- Accurately file all paper medical records.
- Check for misfiled records and file them properly.
- Understand the definition of an "inactive" client or patient record. Every six months, remove or "purge" records of patients who meet the inactive status. Store these records numerically or alphabetically as directed.
- Retain a list of inactive clients, and know where inactive files are stored.

General Medical-Record Tasks
- Ensure that medical charts or records to be filed are complete and that they include current laboratory test results, doctors' notes, and forms. Ensure that records have been updated to reflect financial transactions, medications and products dispensed, weights, immunizations, and diagnoses.
- Understand and properly use special record notations, including male, female, aggressive, caution, no credit/charging, and inactive.

- Transfer patient records upon written request of clients and approval of attending doctors or the practice owner.

Reception-Area and Front-Office Tasks

Front-Office Management Tasks

- Schedule receptionists in a manner that meets the practice's and staff's needs.
- Assist in the hiring of new receptionists by advising candidates of openings, offering them applications, working with them to help evaluate their personalities and skill levels, and providing your opinion to the hiring manager.
- Train new receptionists in the basic skills of the position and the practice's philosophy.
- Train receptionists in the areas where they need to expand their skills and knowledge.
- Repair malfunctioning equipment or bring the malfunction to the manager's attention.

Reception-Area Housekeeping Tasks

- Keep the reception area clean and organized by dusting, picking up trash, and organizing the work area.
- Vacuum or sweep the reception area and waiting room as needed to keep these areas clean and free of hair.
- Place mats on the floor and towels by the door on rainy or snowy days to prevent clients and patients from slipping and to minimize the tracking in of water and mud.
- Offer towels to pet owners to dry their pets during inclement weather.
- Clean urinary and fecal accidents in the waiting room immediately; check with doctors or technicians to see if they need samples for diagnostics before discarding them.
- Maintain a current and attractive selection of reading material in the reception area.
- Check exam rooms between clients and straighten them as needed by sweeping, cleaning the exam table and instruments, and restocking rooms. Dispose of used needles and syringes as set forth by the practice's policy and OSHA standards.

- Check public restroom(s) and clean them as needed. Restock toilet paper, paper towels, and hand soap as needed.
- Keep the entrance, stairs, and sidewalks clean, safe, and presentable.
- Keep coffee and beverages stocked and available for clients.
- Turn on the radio or sound system at the beginning of the day, and turn it off at the end of the day.
- Keep the temperature at a comfortable level. As established by the practice manager, adjust the heat or air-conditioning as needed. Ensure that windows are closed when the air-conditioning is on.
- Water, feed, and maintain plants so that they are vibrant and add to the professional appearance of the practice.

SUPPLIES-MANAGEMENT TASKS

- Restock office supplies and products in the retail and pharmacy areas.
- Establish and/or maintain a list of depleted office supplies, handouts, and medical-record supplies. Order replacement supplies or request that the office manager do so.
- Keep forms, brochures, and handouts neatly stocked and readily available to share with clients.
- Assist with drug, food, and supply inventory management by following inventory-management protocols and notifying manager(s) of low stock.
- Receive deliveries; check contents of deliveries against invoices and immediately note package shortages or damaged shipments.

OTHER RECEPTION-AREA TASKS

- Maintain the bulletin board or showcase information in an orderly and attractive format.
- Maintain contact with animal-control officers, animal inspectors, and town officials regarding lost or stray animals and animals subject to rabies quarantines.
- Maintain a file of lost and found pets.
- Maintain a phone and address list of local resources for training, boarding, and grooming, as well as for animal-control officers, animal inspectors, city officials, township officials, state officials, veterinary medical association contacts, and other professional contacts.

- Set up referral appointments and complete all necessary paperwork.
- Label and mail monthly service reminders in a timely fashion.
- Be prepared to handle medical emergencies at all times. Recognize the symptoms of pets and clients in crisis. Alert doctors and technicians to emergency situations. Prepare rooms for incoming emergencies.
- Follow scheduling guidelines to maximize efficiency when booking clients. Properly utilize emergency or open slots in the schedule.
- Reorganize daily appointment schedules as needed to account for emergency situations and time overruns.
- Follow isolation procedures when greeting clients with contagious or potentially contagious patients. Using the designated products and dilutions for disinfectants, properly disinfect your shoes, hands, and clothing before leaving isolation areas.
- Assign and dispense rabies tags.
- Send correspondence, including thank-you notes, condolence cards, and welcome cards.

Computer Tasks

General Computer Tasks

- Use your own password identification to enter the practice-management software and signify your work.
- Properly use the doctor's identification to attribute work performed by various doctors to their production records.
- Print appointment, drop-off, and surgery schedules for each day.
- Print a list of expected boarders and grooming clients for each day.
- Schedule examinations, drop-offs, surgery, grooming appointments, and boarding reservations.
- Use practice-management software procedures to check in clients.
- Back up computer files at the close of each business day or as directed.
- Know the clip-art and desktop-publishing software sufficiently to develop or aid in the development of forms, notices, and newsletters.

Database-Management Tasks

- Add new clients and new patients into the computer system as appropriate.
- Inactivate clients or patients using correct software procedures.
- Insert notes regarding important communications with clients in computerized or hard-copy medical records.
- Enter notes, diagnoses, and/or travel-sheet diagnostic codes from doctors regarding examination findings, treatments, diagnostics, procedures, and diagnoses.
- Inquire about and record vital changes in client or patient information, including weight, immunization status, microchip number, and spay/neuter status. Update the medical record in the computer.
- Input reminders and callbacks.

Word-Processing Tasks

- Know the word-processing program sufficiently to draft letters and modify and print forms or letters.
- Print hard copies of forms for incoming clients whose pets will have anesthetic, surgical, dental, or medical procedures.
- Generate records of rabies immunizations for clients and town, city, and county officials.
- Produce immunization, health, and neuter certificates.

Report-Generation Tasks

- Print monthly service reminders.
- Create daily callback list(s) and transfer them to person(s) responsible for calls.
- Generate end-of-day reports.
- Generate end-of-month reports and end-of-year reports.
- Adjust computerized products and supplies inventory to reflect items used and/or disposed of.
- Search for, save, and print special lists from the database, such as patients that are overdue for services, new patients, and/or new clients per month.

Internet-Based Tasks

- Know how to access and navigate the Internet to download email, find veterinary websites, order supplies, and access information for clients.
- Be familiar with the practice's website.
- Prepare and send email reminders and notices.
- Respond to basic questions sent via email.
- Handle online appointment bookings.

Financial Tasks

Cash-Management Tasks

- Ensure that the cash register has sufficient change for each day's monetary transactions. Change money at the bank as necessary.
- Count and record the cash in the drawer each morning and at shift changes.
- Count and record the cash in the drawer at closing. Reduce the drawer to the starting amount of cash.

Daily Closing Financial Tasks

- Prepare daily bank deposits.
- Ask the practice manager or owner to deliver deposits to the bank on a daily basis.
- Balance the daily and monthly revenue records against check deposits and credit and cash receipts; check math for accuracy.
- Match each day's monetary intake (cash, checks, and credit cards slips) with the computerized day summary sheet or handwritten invoices.

Payment-Processing Tasks

- Correctly apply discounts for employees, shelters, multiple pets, coupons, and complimentary exams.

- Properly enter charges from travel or circle sheets or patient records into the computer.
- Process clients' cash, credit card, debit card, and check payments.
- Accurately record all payments in client/patient records and in the bookkeeping system.
- Give accurate change.
- Ensure that checks have proper identifying information recorded on them (identity or driver's license number), that checks are dated and signed, and that clients have provided and you have reviewed proper corroborating identification.
- Process checks properly for electronic check acceptance.
- Check that clients' signatures on credit receipts match those on credit cards or their photo identification.
- Provide clients with printed receipts of their transactions, whether or not they have requested them.
- Produce legible and accurate receipts.
- Review itemized entries on receipts with clients at the time of payment.
- Answer clients' questions regarding charges, or refer questions to the appropriate colleague.

Tasks Related to Incomplete Payments

- Process and help clients complete CareCredit® applications.
- Complete or file pet health insurance claims on behalf of clients as directed by the practice manager or doctors.
- Process clients' credit applications and store them in clients' records.
- Properly record and file deferred payments.
- Record returned checks and adjust clients' accounts to reflect returned-check fees.
- Issue updated invoices to clients, including appropriate finance charges, and show accurate balances due on their accounts.
- Search for and refer delinquent accounts to a collection service as directed by the practice manager.

CHAPTER 3

RECEPTIONIST TRAINING SCHEDULE

Week One

By the end of week one, new receptionists should have learned to:

General Knowledge and Tasks

- Know the range of services the practice provides and the species it treats.
- Follow OSHA standards. Be able to find Material Safety Data Sheets quickly.
- Maintain accurate personal time cards.

Client-Interaction Tasks

- Advise clients of special call-in times to check on patients or speak with doctors.
- Escort clients and patients to clean, empty exam rooms free of persistent, offensive odors.
- Assist clients with unruly or unrestrained pets. Ensure that all dogs are leashed and that cats and smaller pets are caged. Isolate aggressive pets. Request assistance if needed.
- Seek the assistance of doctors or technicians immediately when assessing potentially critical patients.

General Telephone Tasks

- Answer the phone by the third ring and use the recommended greeting.

- Know phone functions, including hold, intercom, transfer, forward, and three-way calling.
- Follow the written telephone scripts.
- Transfer calls to the answering service or set the answering machine to accept calls during staff meetings and hours when the practice is closed. Stop the transfer of calls to service or turn off the answering machine when staff members are available to receive calls.

Medical-Record Management Tasks

- Pull charts for incoming clients.
- Check for and enter phone, address, and email updates in clients' records and medical updates (spay/neuter status, immunization status, microchip number) in patients' records.
- Properly use bins or slots assigned to doctors, staff, pharmacy, lab, and callbacks.
- Accurately file all paper medical records.
- Check for misfiled records and file them properly.

Reception-Area and Front-Office Tasks

- Keep the reception area clean and organized by dusting, picking up trash, and organizing the work area.
- Vacuum or sweep the reception area and waiting room as needed to keep these areas clean and free of hair.
- Clean urinary and fecal accidents in the waiting room immediately; check with doctors or technicians to see if they need samples for diagnostics before discarding them.
- Check exam rooms between clients and straighten them as needed by sweeping, cleaning the exam table and instruments, and restocking rooms.
- Dispose of used needles and syringes as set forth by the practice's policy and OSHA standards.
- Check public restroom(s) and clean them as needed. Restock toilet paper, paper towels, and hand soap as needed.
- Keep coffee and beverages stocked and available for clients.

- Turn on the radio or sound system at the beginning of the day and turn it off at the end of the day.
- Keep the temperature at a comfortable level. Adjust the heat or air-conditioning as needed. Ensure that windows are closed when the air-conditioning is on.

Month One

By the end of month one, new receptionists should have learned to:

General Knowledge and Tasks

- Give directions to the practice.
- Maintain a list of tasks and engage in productive work during slow periods.

Client-Interaction Tasks

- Review consent forms with clients and have clients sign the forms. Check that clients' signatures match the signatures on the records.
- Using reminder, recall-system, and outpatient-visit and patient-admission protocols, advise clients of recommended services for their pets.
- Explain delays that affect clients. Ensure the comfort of clients and patients. Reschedule appointments as needed.
- Explain special programs offered by the practice.
- Provide clients with handouts and brochures regarding relevant medical conditions, surgeries, immunizations, internal and external parasites, pet insurance, and diets.
- Discharge hospitalized patients and boarded and groomed pets. Review discharge instructions and medications with clients. Give a copy of the instructions to the client and put a copy in the medical record. Discuss any problems noted in the record. For hospitalized patients, schedule recheck (medical-progress) appointments and follow-up callbacks.

- Provide clients with information regarding options available for the remains of deceased pets.
- Distribute puppy, kitten, and new patient kits.
- Schedule appointments for exams, rechecks, surgeries, medical procedures, boarding, and grooming.
- Call clients with hospitalized pets to provide patient-status updates.
- Provide basic pricing information to callers. Respond in a manner that encourages potential clients to visit the practice.
- Receive and record prescription-refill requests.
- Schedule euthanasias to maximize the comfort of clients and patients while allowing the practice to run efficiently.
- Schedule house calls according to written guidelines.
- Call clients scheduled for the next day to remind them of their appointments, appointment times, and special instructions, such as the need for fasting or withholding or administering medications.
- Call clients on callback lists to check on patients' well-being and answer questions.
- Call clients who missed appointments and reschedule their appointments.
- Obtain current patient-status reports or updates from doctors, technicians, or assistants.

General Telephone Tasks

- Transcribe messages from the answering machine and distribute messages appropriately.
- Accurately record messages for doctors and staff. Note the caller's name, date, time of call, return phone number, and message. Notify the recipient of an urgent message immediately. Place routine messages in appropriate boxes.

Medical-Record Management Tasks

- Upon the client's arrival, mark the patient's medical record with the date and a brief synopsis of the reasons for the visit.
- Attach a travel or circle sheet marked with the patient's and client's names to the medical record of each arriving client.

- For patients that are being admitted, attach cage cards and completed client-consent or other forms to the records.
- Understand the medical-record filing system.
- Know all possible locations for storage of records of hospitalized patients.
- Understand and use special record notations, including male, female, aggressive, caution, no credit/charging, and inactive.

Reception-Area and Front-Office Tasks

- Understand emergency procedures so that they can be implemented immediately in case of fire, theft, dangerous persons, or the presence of unrestrained pets.
- Restock office supplies and products in the retail and pharmacy areas.
- Establish and/or maintain a list of depleted office supplies, handouts, and medical-record supplies. Order replacement supplies or request that the office manager do so.
- Keep forms, brochures, and handouts neatly stocked and readily available to share with clients.
- Assist with drug, food, and supply inventory management by following inventory-management protocols and notifying manager(s) of low stock.
- Follow scheduling guidelines to maximize efficiency when booking clients. Properly utilize emergency or open slots in the schedule.
- Reorganize daily appointment schedules as needed to account for emergency situations and time overruns.
- Follow isolation procedures when greeting clients with contagious or potentially contagious patients. Using the designated products and dilutions for disinfectants, properly disinfect your shoes, hands, and clothing before leaving isolation areas.
- Assign and dispense rabies tags.

Computer Tasks

- Properly use your own password identification to enter the practice-management software and signify your work.

- Properly use doctor identification to attribute work performed by various doctors to their production records.
- Print appointment, drop-off, and surgery schedules for each day.
- Print a list of expected boarders and grooming clients for each day.
- Schedule examinations, drop-offs, surgery, grooming appointments, and boarding reservations.
- Use practice-management software procedures to check in clients.
- Back up computer files at the close of each business day or as directed.
- Add new clients and new patients into the computer system as appropriate.
- Insert notes regarding important communications with clients in computerized or hard-copy medical records.
- Enter notes, diagnoses, and/or travel-sheet diagnostic codes from doctors regarding examination findings, treatments, diagnostics, and diagnoses into the computer system.
- Inquire about and record vital changes in client or patient information and update the medical record in the computer.
- Input reminders and callbacks.
- Produce immunization, health, and neuter certificates.
- Generate end-of-day reports.
- Be familiar with the practice's website.

Financial Tasks

- Count and record the cash in the drawer each morning and at shift changes.
- Count and record the cash in the drawer at closing. Reduce the drawer to the starting amount of cash.
- Balance the daily and monthly revenue records against check deposits and credit and cash receipts; check math for accuracy.
- Match each day's monetary intake (cash, checks, and credit card slips) with the computerized day summary sheet or handwritten invoices.
- Process clients' cash, credit card, debit card, and check payments.

- Accurately record all payments in client/patient records and into the bookkeeping system.
- Process checks properly for electronic check acceptance.
- Provide clients with printed receipts of their transactions, whether or not they have requested them.
- Properly enter charges from travel or circle sheets or patient records into the computer.
- Produce legible and accurate receipts.
- Review itemized entries on receipts with clients at the time of payment.
- Answer clients' questions regarding charges or refer questions to the appropriate colleague.

Month Three

By the end of month three, new receptionists should have learned to:

General Knowledge and Tasks

- Be reasonably familiar with breeds and coat colors.
- Know standard medical and business abbreviations.
- Understand the life cycle and pathology of common parasites (intestinal parasites, heartworms, fleas, ticks), and know the names of most common preventatives, recommended treatments, and diagnostics.
- Be familiar with zoonotic (contagious) diseases, including their prevention and steps to reduce or eliminate transmission.
- Communicate with clients about the various pet-identification systems available, including tags, tattoos, and microchips.
- Know the policies regarding provision of veterinary care, treatment of stray animals, deposits for hospitalized patients, payments, credit, pet health insurance, and finance fees.
- Participate in your performance appraisal, and, as requested, in those of others.

CLIENT-INTERACTION TASKS

- Provide clients with accurate and thorough information about all over-the-counter products sold at the practice. Understand and explain internal and external parasite products as well as diets, dental products, and behavior management tools.
- Give estimates for services to be performed on patients.
- Dispense prescribed medications and diets to clients. Discuss dosing and administration instructions to ensure that clients understand the use of prescribed products. Advise clients of common side effects of dispensed medications as instructed by doctors or technicians.
- Answer routine questions or refer calls to appropriate colleagues.
- Verify and obtain approval from a veterinarian prior to dispensing or delivering medication to a client.
- Prepare medications and prescriptions for dispensing as directed by the doctor. Ensure that each prescription label contains the following information: doctor's name; practice's name, address, and phone number including area code; date; patient's and client's name; medication name, strength and volume (or number); administration instructions including route of administration, such as by mouth or in the ear; and product's expiration date.

GENERAL TELEPHONE TASKS

- Manage multiple phone lines effectively; prioritize phone calls.
- Call in prescriptions to outside pharmacies.

RECEPTION-AREA AND FRONT-OFFICE TASKS

- Follow established closing procedures to ensure the security of patients, staff, data, revenue, inventory, and the facility.
- Receive deliveries; check contents of deliveries against invoices and immediately note package shortages or damaged shipments.

Computer Tasks

- Print hard copies of forms for incoming patients that will undergo anesthetic, surgical, dental, or medical procedures.
- Generate estimates from standard estimates or doctors' estimates.

Financial Tasks

- Prepare daily bank deposits.
- Understand options and correctly apply discounts for employees, shelters and multiple pets, coupons, and complimentary exams.
- Process and help clients complete CareCredit® applications.
- Process clients' credit applications and store them in clients' records.

Month Six

By the end of month six, new receptionists should have learned to:

General Knowledge and Tasks

- Use proper medical terminology when speaking and writing.

Client-Interaction Tasks

- Advise clients of significant changes in the policies or services since their last visit.
- Handle angry or grieving clients in a calm, reassuring manner. Escort complaining or angry clients from the reception area to a separate, closed room where their complaints may be heard privately. When necessary, enlist a doctor or the office manager to resolve the complaint.

- Placate and/or compensate clients distressed by long waits, scheduling glitches, or other problems.
- Provide basic grief counseling or arrange for more in-depth counseling for clients in need.
- Conduct tours of the practice and/or kennel. Before each tour, ensure that the facility is orderly and that staff and patients are prepared for tours.

Medical-Record Management Tasks

- Understand the definition of an "inactive" client or patient record. Every six months, remove or "purge" records of patients who meet the inactive status. Store these records numerically or alphabetically as directed.
- Retain a list of inactive clients, and know where inactive files are stored.
- Ensure that records to be filed are complete and that they include current laboratory test results, doctors' notes, and forms. Ensure that patient records have been updated to reflect financial transactions, medications and products dispensed, weights, immunizations, and diagnoses.
- Transfer patient records upon written requests of clients and the approval of attending doctors or the practice owner.

Reception-Area and Front-Office Tasks

- Assist in the hiring of new receptionists by advising candidates of openings, offering them applications, working with them to help evaluate their personalities and skill levels, and providing your opinion to the hiring manager.
- Repair malfunctioning equipment or bring the malfunction to the manager's attention.
- Maintain the bulletin board or showcase information in an orderly and attractive format.
- Maintain contact with animal-control officers, animal inspectors, and town officials regarding lost or stray animals and animals subject to rabies quarantines.

- Maintain a file of lost and found pets.
- Maintain a phone and address list of local resources for training, boarding, and grooming, as well as for animal-control officers, animal inspectors, city officials, township officials, state officials, veterinary medical association contacts, and other professional contacts.
- Set up referral appointments and complete all necessary paperwork.
- Label and mail monthly service reminders in a timely fashion.
- Be prepared to handle medical emergencies at all times. Recognize the symptoms of pets and clients in crisis. Alert doctors and technicians to emergency situations. Prepare rooms for incoming emergencies.
- Send correspondence, including thank-you notes, condolence cards, and welcome cards.

Computer Tasks

- Know the clip-art and desktop publishing software sufficiently to develop or aid in the development of forms, notices, and newsletters.
- Inactivate clients or patients using correct software procedures.
- Know the word-processing program sufficiently to draft letters and modify and print forms or letters.
- Generate records of rabies vaccines for clients and town/city/county officials.
- Print monthly service reminders.
- Generate daily callback list(s) and transfer them to the person(s) responsible for calls.
- Generate end-of-month reports and end-of-year reports.
- Adjust the computerized products and supplies inventory to reflect items used and/or dispensed.
- Search for, save, and print special lists from the database, such as patients that are overdue for services, new patients, and/or new clients per month.
- Know how to access and navigate the Internet to download email, find veterinary websites, order supplies, and access information for clients.
- Prepare and send email reminders and notices.

- Respond to basic questions sent via email.
- Handle online appointment bookings.

Financial Tasks

- Ensure that the cash register has sufficient change for each day's monetary transactions. Change money at the bank as necessary.
- Complete or file pet-insurance claims on behalf of clients as directed by the practice manager or doctors.
- Properly record and file deferred payments.
- Record returned checks and adjust the client accounts to reflect returned-check fees.
- Issue updated invoices to clients, including appropriate finance charges, and show accurate balances due on their accounts.
- Search for and refer delinquent accounts to a collection service as directed by the practice manager.

CHAPTER 4

VETERINARY ASSISTANT JOB DESCRIPTION

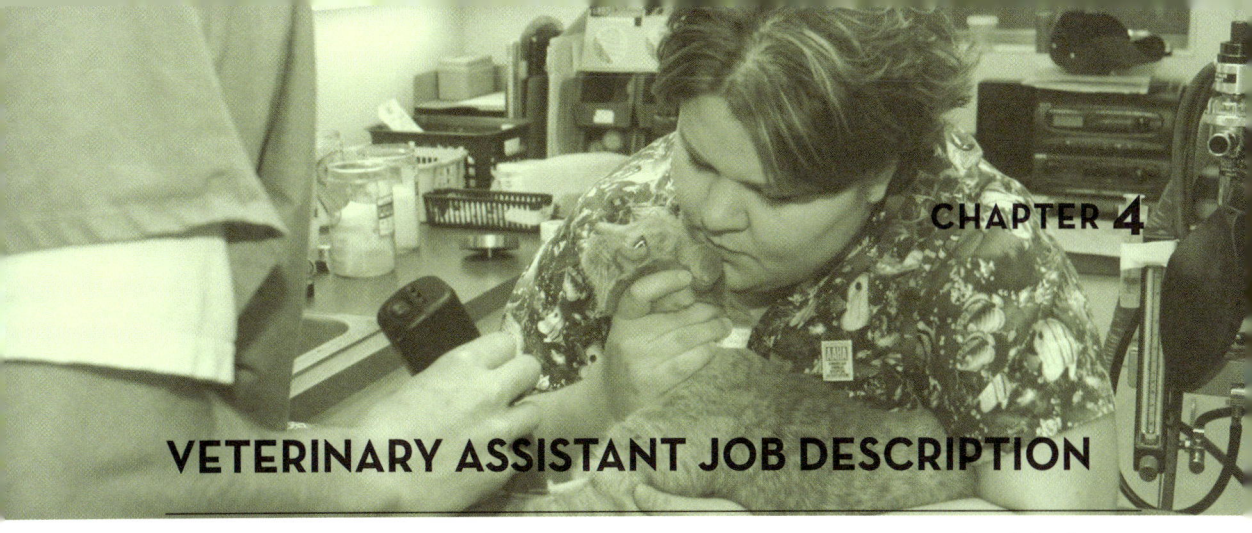

The responsibilities of veterinary assistants vary considerably from one practice to another. In some situations, they may be assigned to assist only in the exam room or to assist only the veterinary technicians. More typically, though, they will divide their time between assisting the receptionists, helping doctors with physical examinations, dispensing medications, and helping veterinary technicians position patients for and process radiographs, prepare patients for surgery, provide nursing and comfort care, and perform treatments or basic laboratory diagnostic tests.

Veterinary assistants must build positive, professional relationships with clients and staff members. Assistants should have completed or be in the process of completing their high school diplomas and must pursue significant on-the-job training.

General Knowledge and Tasks

General Knowledge

- Give directions to the practice.
- Know the range of services the practice provides and the species it treats.
- Be reasonably familiar with breeds and coat colors.
- Follow OSHA standards. Be able to find Material Safety Data Sheets quickly.
- Know and use standard medical and business abbreviations.
- Use proper medical terminology when speaking and writing.
- Understand the life cycle and pathology of common parasites (intestinal parasites, heartworms, fleas, ticks), and know the names of most common preventatives, recommended treatments, and diagnostics.
- Be familiar with zoonotic (contagious) diseases, including their prevention and steps to reduce or eliminate transmission.

- Know the policies regarding provision of veterinary care, treatment of stray animals, deposits for hospitalized patients, payments, credit, pet health insurance, and finance fees.
- Competently speak and write the English language.
- Competently speak a second language commonly used at the practice.

General Tasks

- Always be in position and prepared to work by the start of each scheduled shift.
- Maintain accurate personal time cards.
- Enter the practice through the front door so that you see what clients see. Routinely pick up trash or feces from the parking lot, sidewalks, or entryway.
- Maintain a professional appearance while at work, including clean and pressed uniforms or clothes. Change clothes daily as necessary to look professional and avoid carrying odors.
- Smile and maintain an even, friendly demeanor while on the job.
- Perform job tasks efficiently without rushing.
- Promote a positive attitude among staff.
- Handle stress and pressure with poise and tact.
- Be willing and available to stay late or through breaks, when needed, to assist with emergency or critical-care patients.
- Show respect for clients, team members, and animals (alive or deceased) at all times.
- Effectively promote preventive health care, nutrition, and pet health insurance to clients. Support what fellow staff members have said to clients.
- Have the physical strength and ability to stand for an entire shift when needed, and be able to lift pets and objects weighing up to 50 pounds without assistance. Assist in lifting patients weighing more than 50 pounds.
- Maintain a list of tasks and engage in productive work during slow periods.
- Assist other employees as needed. Avoid waiting for coworkers to ask for assistance.
- Stock hospital supplies and pharmaceutical, pet-food, and over-the-counter products.

- Ensure that medical supplies are always available. Add new items to the list of depleted supplies.
- Regularly check for outdated supplies. Remove and replace them as directed by the office manager.
- Assist in hiring new assistants by advising candidates of openings, offering them applications, working with them to help evaluate their personalities and skill levels, and providing your opinion to the hiring manager.
- Participate in your performance appraisal, and, as requested, in those of others.
- Participate in all staff and training meetings.
- Conduct tours of the practice and/or kennel. Before each tour, ensure that the facility is orderly and that staff and patients are prepared for tours.
- Maintain constant vigilance regarding open doorways that could allow pets to escape from the facility.
- Maintain strict confidentiality regarding clients and patients for whom the practice provides veterinary services.
- Be prepared to handle any pet or facility emergency that may arise, including dog or cat fights, choking or strangulating animals, and facility fire or weather-related emergencies. Follow contingency plans.
- Follow established closing procedures to ensure the security of patients, staff, data, revenue, inventory, and the facility.

Front-Office Tasks

- Know phone functions, including hold, intercom, transfer, forward, and three-way calling.
- Answer the phone by the third ring when receptionists are preoccupied or unavailable.
- Assist receptionists in keeping the facility's reception area and room(s) clean and tidy. Replace older issues of magazines with current ones, placed neatly in holders or on tables.
- When assisting at the reception desk, know names of clients and patients that are scheduled to arrive before they appear.
- Access client information within the practice-management software system. Enter and retrieve client and patient data in the computer.

- Assist receptionists with clients' payments, and provide clients with receipts that detail their transactions.

Client-Interaction Tasks

Patient-Admittance Tasks

- Cordially greet incoming clients and patients, addressing each by name.
- Check clients in. Update clients' or patients' records as needed.
- Use clients' and patients' names during conversations.
- Counsel clients on financial and admittance policies, their pets' medical procedures, and options that require consideration. Answer clients' questions and ensure that all admittance paperwork is properly completed. Check that clients' signatures on consent forms match those on new client information sheets.
- Advise clients of special call-in times to check on patients or speak with doctors.
- Inform clients of recommended services for their pets and obedience training or special health care programs offered by the practice.
- Provide clients with accurate and thorough information about over-the-counter products. Understand and explain internal and external parasite products as well as diets, dental products, and behavior management tools.
- Know where brochures and client-education materials are stored. Provide clients with handouts and brochures regarding relevant medical conditions, surgeries, immunizations, internal and external parasites, pet insurance, and diets.
- Give estimates for services to be performed on patients.
- Advise clients of significant changes in policies or services since their last visit.
- Explain delays that affect clients. Ensure the comfort of clients and patients during their waits. Offer water to clients or patients in need (or withhold water from patients as appropriate). Reschedule appointments as needed.
- Call for waiting clients using pets' names and clients' last names. Lead them to exam rooms.

- Transfer incoming patients to appropriate wards and ensure the comfort of clients and patients. Identify patients with cage cards and/or neck bands. Add patients to each day's census, procedure list, or surgery schedule.
- Assist clients with unruly or unrestrained pets. When assisting receptionists, ensure that all dogs are leashed immediately after arrival and that cats and smaller pets are caged. Isolate aggressive pets. Request assistance if needed.

Pet-Identification Tasks

- Scan new patients and strays for microchips, tags, and tattoos. Identify and record microchip numbers, tattoos, and/or patient markings in patients' records.
- Communicate with clients about the various pet-identification systems available, including tags, tattoos, and microchips.
- Assist clients in registering pet-identification information in the practice's computer system and in the appropriate national database.

Patient-Discharge Tasks

- Coordinate patient transfers with front desk, kennel and/or veterinarians.
- Prepare medications and prescriptions for dispensing as directed by the doctor. Ensure that each prescription label contains the following information: doctor's name; practice's name, address, and phone number including area code; date; patient's and client's name; medication name, strength and volume (or number); administration instructions including route of administration, such as by mouth or in the ear; and product's expiration date.
- Dispense medications. Discuss administration or application of products and potential side effects with owners as instructed by doctors or technicians.
- Provide clients with accurate and thorough information about all over-the-counter products. Understand and explain internal- and external-parasite products as well as diets, dental products, and behavior management tools.
- Accurately invoice clients from charges on travel or circle sheets or medical records.

- Discharge patients. Instruct clients on the care of patients at home, timing of recheck appointments, and potential adverse effects of surgeries, procedures, or medications.
- Assist grieving clients and comfort them. Be familiar with the grieving process. Always be sensitive to background chatter or conversations that could exacerbate the anxieties and grief clients experience during euthanasias or deaths of their pets.
- Provide clients with memorials of their dead-on-arrival, died-during-hospitalization, or euthanized pets, (e.g., locks of hair, paw prints, or paw molds). Return collars, leashes, and other accessories.
- Handle angry or grieving clients in a calm, reassuring manner. Escort complaining or angry clients from the reception area to a separate, closed room where their complaints may be heard privately. When necessary, enlist a doctor or the office manager to resolve the complaint.
- Assist clients to their cars if needed.

Medical-Record Management Tasks

- Understand the medical-record filing system.
- Know all possible locations for storage of records of hospitalized patients.
- Locate medical files for hospitalized, surgical, or incoming patients.
- Check on the immunizations or reminder status of arriving pets.
- Properly use bins or slots assigned to doctors, staff, pharmacy, lab, and callbacks.
- Attach a travel or circle sheet marked with the patient's and client's names to the medical record of each arriving client.
- For patients being admitted to the facility, attach cage cards and completed client forms to the records.
- Understand and use special record notations, including male, female, aggressive, caution, no credit/charging, and/or inactive.
- Record doctors' and technicians' notes in patients' computer records or on paper records.
- Make notes in patients' files of relevant phone or in-person conversations with clients, and place your initials after such entries.

- Verify and/or witness clients' statements regarding procedures, including euthanasias.
- Check files for completeness of notes, charges, callbacks, and reminders before refiling. Ensure that records include current laboratory tests, procedure results, current patients' weights, immunizations, diagnoses, and treatments.
- Accurately file all paper medical records.

Exam-Room Tasks

- Possess sufficient strength and assertiveness to effectively restrain patients and ensure the safety of clients and personnel.
- Clean and straighten exam rooms to prepare for incoming patients. Spray disinfectant on exam tables, wipe them clean, and dry them. Remove sources of offensive odors; empty trash if necessary. Check floors, walls, doors, and counters, and sweep or clean them as needed to remove hair, body fluids, and dirt.
- Measure and record each patient's weight, temperature, pulse rate, and respiratory rate.
- Answer questions and educate clients about basic pet care and procedures including nutrition; internal and external parasite control; immunization protocols; the administration of topical, oral, otic, and ophthalmic medications; spay and neuter procedures; and behavior and training. Refer questions you cannot answer to appropriate colleagues.
- Using aseptic procedures, draw up vaccines and/or injections that doctors will administer.
- Administer vaccines subcutaneously and intramuscularly. Follow the practice's policies, the manufacturers' directions, and AAFP guidelines for the placement of vaccines.
- Dispose of used needles and syringes and other sharp objects as set forth by the practice's policy and OSHA standards.
- Perform suture removals, nail trims, and wing trims.
- Assist with routine exam-room procedures, such as venipunctures, skin scrapings, fine-needle aspirates, corneal stains, and ear treatments.
- Lay out and/or set up instruments that doctors will use during ophthalmic, otic, oral, and/or skin examinations, as determined

by the patients' presenting complaints, prior to the doctors' arrivals in rooms.
- Take photographs or videos of patients' conditions and lesions as directed by veterinarians.
- Record doctors' findings during medical examinations.
- Keep a small notebook or personal digital assistant (PDA) in your pocket to record accurate instructions, particularly regarding the preparation and administering medications to be dispensed.
- Keep exam rooms stocked with syringes, needles, bandage materials, and prepackaged dispensable products. Regularly restock exam rooms or pharmacy refrigerators with vaccines.
- Inform the practice manager or doctors immediately of all bite or scratch wounds you suffer so that reports can be made and you can be referred for timely medical care by a physician if necessary. Clean all wounds quickly and thoroughly.

Nursing-Care Tasks

Basic Patient-Care Tasks
- Prioritize tasks to maximize clients' satisfaction and patients' health.
- Track and use or store comfort items brought by clients for hospitalized patients.
- Wash, dry, and store patients' bedding and the practice's towels. Maintain bedding in good repair.
- Place clean, soft bedding in cages as appropriate.
- Maximize patients' comfort with a gentle and reassuring manner. Understand that actions that would constitute animal cruelty under state or local laws or the practice's policies will be grounds for immediate reprimand and/or termination.
- Monitor patients for vomit, blood, urine, and feces in the cage, and clean patients and cages as needed. Save debris if unsure whether it should be examined. Note unexpected incidents on cage cards or charts.
- Monitor patients' behaviors and note potentially aggressive behaviors. Use caution when handling aggressive or potentially aggressive pets. Request assistance when needed.

- Monitor changes in patients' conditions. Alert doctors or technicians to significant changes.
- Follow isolation procedures. Prevent contact between contagious animals and others. Using the designated products and dilutions for disinfectants, properly disinfect your shoes, hands, and clothing before leaving isolation areas.
- Walk dogs on a double leash or on a leash within a fenced exercise area. Ensure that they are restrained and under your control at all times.
- Prepare meals and feed animals. Note appetite on cage cards or patient records.
- Assess hospitalized patients' temperatures, pulse rates, respiratory rates, and respiratory qualities, and record data in appropriate records.
- Deflea patients with flea combs, flea sprays, spot-on topicals, baths, dips, or appropriate medication.
- Detick patients using proper instruments or techniques.
- Provide medical grooming, including medicated baths, dips, and mat removal.
- Clip hair in a manner that minimizes clipper burn. Maintain clean clipper blades and lubricate them on a regular basis.
- Use warning stickers and notations on cage cards and records as appropriate.
- Prior to discharge, remove patients' catheters, clean patients so that no body fluids are detectable, and bathe and/or groom patients prior to transferring them to clients.
- Disinfect cages as soon as possible after patients are removed from them.

Patient-Treatment Tasks
- Understand the mechanics and application of basic standards of asepsis.
- Maintain IV catheters so fluids flow freely; flush and clean as needed.
- Administer IV, IM, SQ, and oral medications and note in charts.
- Assist in the application of wound dressings and treatments.
- Swab, clean, flush, and treat ear canals without causing trauma.
- Trim nails to the quick without causing bleeding.

- Understand how to stop bleeding by using styptic pencils, powder, or other means.
- Monitor and maintain urinary collection bags. Record urine production on cage cards and in charts.
- Identify a patient's level of pain and possible causes of pain, and understand the medications and methods used to control pain.
- Assist kennel staff in medicating and treating boarders.

Technical Tasks

General Technical Tasks

- Restrain pets in a manner that allows necessary work to be performed, minimizes stress to patients, and ensures the safety of patients and people. Safely and effectively apply and use restraints such as muzzles, towels, gloves, and cat bags.
- Perform venipunctures using patients' cephalic, saphenous, and jugular veins in a manner that minimizes trauma to patients and injury to veins and allows you to successfully obtain a non-hemolyzed sample.
- Collect urine and fecal samples. Use fecal loops for stool collection as needed.
- Prepare slides of body fluids. Air dry and stain them as directed.
- Make blood smears with properly feathered edges that ensure accurate white and red blood cell interpretation.
- Maintain stains and other supplies in a manner that avoids contamination and ensures correct results.
- Use proper stain techniques to maximize diagnostic interpretation of prepared slides.
- Maintain test kits under proper environmental conditions.
- Understand the paperwork and procedures of outside laboratories used by the practice.
- Perform routine ELISA tests, such as heartworm and feline viral tests. Set up and read urine specific gravities, hemocrits, and total protein tests.
- Perform fecal examinations, including direct, centrifugation, and flotation procedures.
- Set up and read Azostix®, blood glucose test strips, and urinalysis dipsticks.

- Assist with euthanasia procedures. Hold off veins and release pressure at the appropriate times.

Emergency-Care Tasks

- Apply temporary bandages or splints.
- Provide basic life support, including CPR, airway maintenance, and oxygen therapy.
- Control bleeding using pressure bandages and tourniquets.
- Provide cooling baths and/or enemas for heatstroke patients.

Surgical-Assistance Tasks

- Know the names of instruments and where they are stored.
- Prepare the surgery suite(s) for incoming patients.
- Bring surgical patients to the surgical prep area. Ensure that you have the correct patients by checking cage cards, affixed identifications, and patients' markings and records.
- Check surgery schedules and patients' records to determine procedures to be performed.
- Assist veterinary technicians in administering preoperative medications.
- Under the direction of doctors or technicians, prepare patients for surgery. Trim nails. Clip surgical fields with straight margins. Minimize tissue trauma. Properly scrub and prepare surgical fields. Maintain clean fields when moving patients.
- Attach cardiac and respiratory monitors, pulse oximeters, or ECG monitors to anesthetized patients.
- Properly position and align patients for surgery.
- Use circulating water baths and/or hot-water bottles to maintain the body temperatures of surgical and dental patients.
- Ground patients when using electrocautery.
- Assist surgeons with aseptic gowning and gloving.
- Wear personal dosimeters as recommended by dosimeter provider.
- Monitor patients during surgery for depth of anesthesia, color, temperature, respiratory rate, and heart rate. Alert doctors to changes in condition.

- Monitor patients' recovery. Protect patients from aspiration and hypothermia. Deflate cuffs and remove endotracheal tubes as soon as gag reflexes return.

SURGICAL CLEANING TASKS

- Clean operating rooms and equipment after use.
- Clean floors and counters in surgical prep and recovery areas, treatment rooms, and wards after use and as needed.
- Wash, sterilize, and store endotracheal tubes using techniques that prevent the spread of disease.
- Clean surgical instruments by hand and/or ultrasonic cleaner.
- Operate and maintain the autoclave.
- Pack and autoclave instruments. Using lists of instruments or photos as guides, ensure that packs contain the proper numbers and types of instruments and that they are labeled with dates and types of packs. Apply pressure and temperature sterilization tape and/or monitors, and verify effectiveness after autoclaving.

RADIOLOGY TASKS

- Assist veterinary technicians and/or doctors with restraint and positioning of patients for radiographic procedures.
- Minimize radiation hazards. Use protective equipment and wear exposure badges whenever exposing radiographs.
- Consistently place right and left markers on cassettes.
- Properly store plates and unexposed film.
- Understand darkroom procedures, including film labeling, film developing, and cassette refilling. Develop film using an automatic processor or by hand processing with tanks. Understand temperature and time variables required for manual processing of radiographs.
- Understand the radiograph filing system. Properly file and/or retrieve films.

CHAPTER 5

VETERINARY ASSISTANT TRAINING SCHEDULE

Week One

By the end of week one, new assistants should have learned to:

General Knowledge and Tasks

- Follow OSHA standards. Be able to find Material Safety Data Sheets quickly.
- Know the policies regarding provision of veterinary care, treatment of stray animals, deposits for hospitalized patients, payments, credit, pet health insurance, and finance fees.
- Maintain accurate personal time cards.
- Participate in their performance appraisals, and, as requested, in those of others.
- Maintain constant vigilance regarding open doorways that could allow pets to escape from the facility.

Front-Office Tasks

- Assist receptionists in keeping the facility's reception area and room(s) clean and tidy. Replace older issues of magazines with current ones, placed neatly in holders or on tables.

Client-Interaction Tasks

- Coordinate patient transfers with front desk, kennel, and/or veterinarians.

Medical-Record Management Tasks

- Understand the medical-record filing system.
- Know all possible locations for storage of records of hospitalized patients.
- Locate medical files for hospitalized, surgical, or incoming patients.
- Properly use bins or slots assigned to doctors, staff, pharmacy, lab, and callbacks.
- Accurately file all paper medical records.

Exam-Room Tasks

- Clean and straighten exam rooms to prepare for incoming patients. Spray disinfectant on exam tables, wipe them clean, and dry them. Remove sources of offensive odors; empty trash if necessary. Check floors, walls, doors, and counters, and sweep or clean as needed to remove hair, body fluids, and dirt.
- Dispose of used needles and syringes and other sharp objects as set forth by the practice's policy and OSHA standards.

Nursing-Care Tasks

- Wash, dry, and store patients' bedding and the practice's towels. Bedding should be in good repair.
- Track and use or store comfort items brought by clients for hospitalized patients.
- Walk dogs on a double leash or on a leash within a fenced exercise area. Ensure that they are restrained and under your control at all times.
- Prepare meals and feed animals. Note appetite on cage cards or patient records.

Month One

By the end of month one, new assistants should have learned to:

General Knowledge and Tasks

- Know and use standard medical and business abbreviations.
- Be familiar with infectious diseases, including their prevention and steps to reduce or eliminate transmission. Know the most common zoonotic diseases (infections from animals to humans).
- Maintain a list of tasks and engage in productive work during slow periods.
- Stock hospital supplies and pharmaceutical, pet-food, and over-the-counter products.
- Ensure that medical supplies are always available. Add new items to the list of depleted supplies.
- Follow established facility closing procedures to ensure the security of patients, staff, data, revenue, inventory, and the building.

Front-Office Tasks

- Know phone functions, including hold, intercom, transfer, forward, and three-way calling.
- Assist receptionists with clients' payments, and provide clients with receipts that detail their transactions.
- Access client information within the practice-management software system. Enter and retrieve client and patient data in the computer.

Client-Interaction Tasks

- Know where brochures and client-education materials are stored. Provide clients with handouts and brochures regarding relevant medical conditions, surgeries, immunizations, internal and external parasites, pet insurance, and diets.
- Assist clients with unruly or unrestrained pets. When assisting receptionists, ensure that all dogs are leashed immediately after arrival and that cats and smaller pets are caged. Isolate aggressive pets. Request assistance if needed.
- Scan new patients and strays for microchips, tags, and tattoos. Identify and record microchip numbers, tattoos, and/or patient markings in patients' records.

- Communicate with clients about the various pet-identification systems available, including tags, tattoos, and microchips.
- Assist clients in registering pet-identification information in the practice's computer system and in the appropriate national database.

Medical-Record Management Tasks

- Understand and use special record notations, including male, female, aggressive, caution, no credit/charging, and/or inactive.
- Record doctors' and technicians' notes in patients' computer records or on paper records.
- Make notes in patients' files of relevant phone or in-person conversations with clients, and place your initials after such entries.
- Verify and/or witness clients' statements regarding procedures, including euthanasias.

Exam-Room Tasks

- Measure and record each patient's weight, temperature, pulse rate, and respiratory rate.
- Using aseptic procedure, draw up vaccines and/or injections doctors will administer.
- Assist with routine exam-room procedures such as venipunctures, skin scrapings, fine-needle aspirates, corneal stains, nail and wing trims, and ear treatments.
- Take photographs or videos of patients' conditions and lesions as directed by veterinarians.
- Record doctors' findings during medical examinations.
- Keep exam rooms stocked with syringes, needles, bandage materials, and prepackaged dispensable products. Regularly restock exam-room or pharmacy refrigerators with vaccines.

Nursing-Care Tasks

- Follow isolation procedures to prevent contact between contagious animals and others. Using the designated products and dilutions for disinfectants, properly disinfect your shoes, hands, and clothing before leaving isolation areas.

- Assess hospitalized patients' temperatures, pulse rates, respiratory rates, and respiratory qualities, and record data in the appropriate records.
- Monitor patients' behaviors and note potentially aggressive behaviors. Use caution when handling aggressive or potentially aggressive pets. Request assistance when needed.
- Deflea patients with flea combs, flea sprays, spot-on topicals, baths, dips, or appropriate medication.
- Detick patients using proper instruments or techniques.
- Provide medical grooming, including medicated baths, dips, nail trims, and mat removal.
- Clip hair in a manner that minimizes clipper burn. Maintain clean clipper blades and lubricate them on a regular basis.
- Use warning stickers and notations on cage cards and records as appropriate.
- Prior to discharge, remove patients' catheters, clean patients so that no body fluids are detectable, and bathe and/or groom them prior to transferring them to clients.
- Trim nails to the quick without causing bleeding.
- Understand how to stop bleeding by using styptic pencils, powder, or other means.
- Identify a patient's level of pain and possible causes of pain, and understand the medications and methods used to control pain.

Technical Tasks

- Restrain pets in a manner that allows necessary work to be performed, minimizes stress to patients, and ensures the safety of patients and people. Safely and effectively apply and use restraints such as muzzles, towels, gloves, and cat bags.
- Maintain test kits under proper environmental conditions.
- Understand the paperwork and procedures of different outside laboratories used by the practice.
- Perform routine ELISA tests, such as heartworm and feline viral tests. Set up and read urine specific gravities, hematocrits, and total protein tests.
- Clean floors and counters in surgical prep and recovery areas, treatment rooms, and wards after use and as needed.

- Wash, sterilize, and store endotracheal tubes using techniques that prevent the spread of disease.
- Clean surgical instruments by hand and/or ultrasonic cleaner.
- Operate and maintain the autoclave.
- Pack and autoclave instruments. Using lists of instruments or photos as guides, ensure that packs contain proper numbers and types of instruments and that they are labeled with dates and types of packs. Apply pressure and temperature sterilization tape and/or monitors and verify effectiveness after autoclaving.
- Assist veterinary technicians and/or doctors with restraint and positioning of patients for radiographic procedures.
- Minimize radiation hazards. Use protective equipment and wear exposure badges whenever exposing radiographs.
- Understand the radiograph filing system. Properly file and/or retrieve films.

Month Three

By the end of month three, new assistants should have learned to:

General Knowledge and Tasks

- Be reasonably familiar with breeds and coat colors.
- Use proper medical terminology when speaking and writing.

Client-Interaction Tasks

- Check clients in. Update clients' or patients' records as needed. Date and note the reasons for clients' visits in medical records.
- Counsel clients on financial and admittance policies, their pets' procedures, and options that require consideration. Answer clients' questions and ensure that all admittance paperwork is properly completed. Check that clients' signatures on consent forms match those on new-client information sheets.
- Advise clients of special call-in times to check on patients or speak with doctors.

- Inform clients of recommended services for their pets and obedience training or special health-care programs offered by the practice.
- Transfer incoming patients to appropriate wards and ensure their comfort. Identify patients with cage cards and/or neck bands. Add patients to each day's census or procedure list or surgery schedule.
- Discharge patients. Instruct clients on the care of patients at home, the timing of recheck appointments, and potential adverse effects of surgeries, procedures, or medications.
- Provide clients with memorials of their dead-on-arrival, died-during-hospitalization, or euthanized pets, (e.g., locks of hair, paw prints, or paw molds). Return collars, leashes, and other accessories.

Medical-Record Management Tasks

- Check on the immunization or other reminder status of arriving pets.
- Attach a travel or circle sheet marked with the patient's and client's names to the medical record of each arriving client.
- For patients being admitted to the facility, attach cage cards and completed client forms to the records.
- Check files for completeness of notes, charges, callbacks, and reminders before refiling. Ensure that records include current laboratory tests, procedure results, current patients' weights, immunizations, diagnoses, and treatments.

Nursing-Care Tasks

- Assist in the application of wound dressings and treatments.
- Monitor and maintain urinary collection bags. Record urine production on cage cards and in charts.

Technical Tasks

- Assist with euthanasia procedures. Hold off veins and release pressure at the appropriate times.
- Control bleeding using pressure bandages and tourniquets.

- Provide cooling baths and/or enemas for heatstroke patients under veterinary supervision.
- Prepare the surgery suite(s) for incoming patients.
- Bring surgical patients to the surgical prep area. Ensure that you have the correct patients by checking cage cards, affixed identification, and patients' markings and records.
- Check surgery schedules and patients' records to determine procedures to be performed.
- Under the direction of doctors or technicians, prepare patients for surgery. Trim nails. Clip surgical fields with straight margins. Minimize tissue trauma. Properly scrub and prepare surgical fields. Maintain clean fields when moving patients.
- Attach cardiac and respiratory monitors, pulse oximeters, or ECG monitors to anesthetized patients.
- Properly position and align patients for surgery.
- Use circulating water baths and/or hot water bottles to maintain the body temperatures of surgical and dental patients.
- Ground patients when using electrocautery.
- Assist surgeons with aseptic gowning and gloving.
- Consistently place right and left markers on cassettes.
- Properly store plates and unexposed film.
- Understand darkroom procedures, including film labeling, film developing, and cassette refilling. Develop film using an automatic processor or by hand processing with tanks. Understand temperature and time variables required for the manual processing of radiographs.

Month Six

By the end of month six, new assistants should have learned to:

General Knowledge and Tasks

- Effectively promote preventive health care, nutrition, and pet health insurance to clients. Support what fellow staff members have said to clients.
- Regularly check for outdated supplies. Remove and replace them as directed by the office manager.

- Assist in hiring new assistants by advising candidates of openings, offering them applications, working with them to help evaluate their personalities and skill levels, and providing your opinion to the hiring manager.
- Conduct tours of the practice and/or kennel. Before each tour, ensure that the facility is orderly and that staff and patients are prepared for tours.

Client-Interaction Tasks

- Provide clients with accurate and thorough information about over-the-counter products. Understand and explain internal- and external-parasite products as well as diets, dental products, and behavior management tools.
- Assist grieving clients and comfort them. Be familiar with the grieving process. Always be sensitive to background chatter or conversations that could disrupt the anxieties and grief clients experience during euthanasias or deaths of their pets.

Exam-Room Tasks

- Answer questions and educate clients about basic pet care and procedures, including nutrition; internal- and external-parasite control; immunization protocols; the administration of topical, oral, otic, and ophthalmic medications; spay and neuter procedures; and behavior and training. Refer questions you cannot answer to appropriate colleagues.
- Administer vaccines subcutaneously and intramuscularly. Follow the practice's policies, manufacturers' directions, and AAFP guidelines for placement of vaccines.
- Perform suture removals, nail trims, and wing trims.
- Lay out and/or set up instruments doctors will use during ophthalmic, otic, oral, and/or skin examinations, as determined by patients' presenting complaints, prior to doctors' arrivals in rooms.

Nursing-Care Tasks

- Monitor changes in patients' conditions. Alert doctors or technicians to significant changes.

- Understand the mechanics and application of basic standards of asepsis.
- Maintain IV catheters so fluids flow freely; flush and clean as needed.
- Administer IV, IM, SQ, and oral medications, and note in charts.
- Swab, clean, flush, and treat ear canals without causing trauma.
- Assist kennel staff in medicating and treating boarders.

Technical Tasks

- Perform venipunctures using patients' cephalic, saphenous, and jugular veins in a manner that minimizes trauma to patients and injury to veins and allows you to successfully obtain a non-hemolyzed sample.
- Collect urine and fecal samples. Use fecal loops for stool collection as needed.
- Prepare slides of body fluids. Air dry and stain them as directed.
- Make blood smears with properly feathered edges that ensure accurate white and red blood cell interpretation.
- Maintain stains and other supplies in a manner that avoids contamination and ensures correct results.
- Use proper stain techniques to maximize diagnostic interpretation of prepared slides.
- Perform fecal examinations, including direct, centrifugation, and flotation procedures.
- Set up and read Azostix®, blood glucose test strips, and urinalysis dipsticks.
- Assist in basic life support, including CPR, airway maintenance, and oxygen therapy.
- Know the names of instruments and where they are stored.
- Wear personal dosimeters as recommended by dosimeter provider.
- Monitor patients during surgery for depth of anesthesia, color, temperature, respiratory rate, and heart rate. Alert doctors to changes in condition.
- Monitor patients' recovery. Protect patients from aspiration and hypothermia. Deflate cuffs and remove endotracheal tubes as soon as gag reflexes return.

CHAPTER 6

VETERINARY TECHNICIAN JOB DESCRIPTION

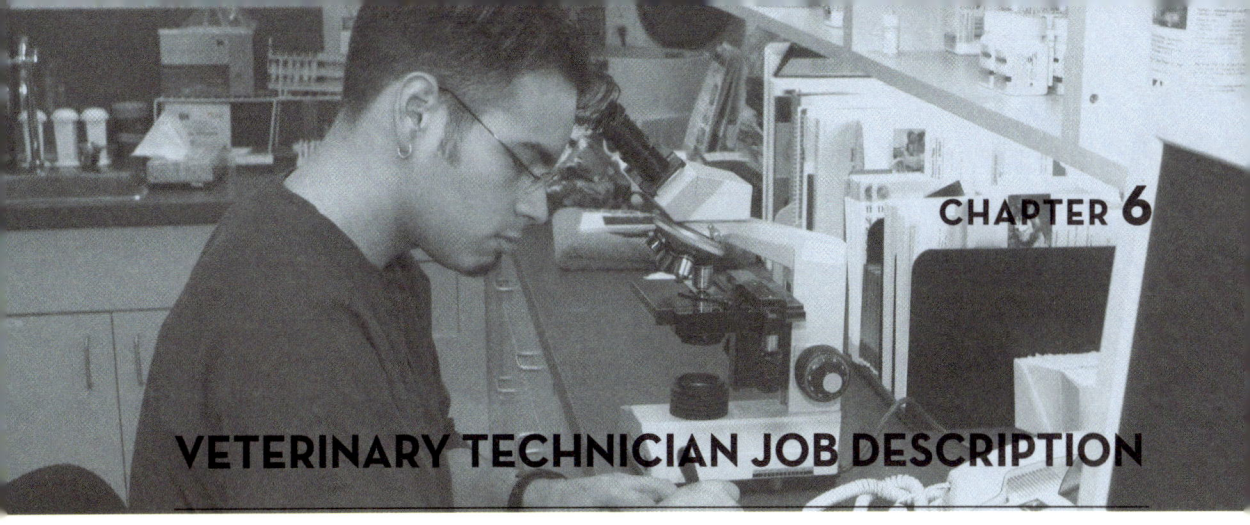

Veterinary technicians may also be identified as registered veterinary technicians, certified veterinary technicians, animal-health technicians, or veterinary nurses. In many states, veterinary technicians are required to have completed an AVMA-accredited veterinary-technician program prior to passing the state's requirements for certification or registration.

Veterinary technicians must have a broad knowledge of animal science, medicine, and husbandry, including a basic knowledge of pharmacology and sufficient mathematical skills to ensure the administration of accurate drug and fluid doses. They must be able to successfully restrain animals, complete clinical laboratory tests, use multiple radiology techniques, administer and monitor animals under anesthesia, assist in surgery, and perform dental procedures. Technicians must also deliver compassionate nursing care.

General Knowledge and Tasks

General Knowledge

- Know the range of services the practice provides and the species it treats.
- Be reasonably familiar with breeds and coat colors.
- Follow OSHA standards. Be able to find Material Safety Data Sheets quickly.
- Know and use standard medical and business abbreviations.
- Use proper medical terminology when speaking and writing.
- Be familiar with infectious diseases, including their prevention and steps to reduce or eliminate transmission. Know the most common zoonotic diseases (infections from animals to humans).
- Competently speak and write the English language.
- Competently speak a second language commonly used at the practice.

General Tasks

- Always be in position and prepared to work at the start of each scheduled shift.
- Maintain accurate personal time cards.
- Enter the practice through the front door so that you see what clients see. Routinely pick up trash or feces from the parking lot, sidewalks, or entryway.
- Maintain a professional appearance while at work, including clean and pressed uniforms or clothes. Change clothes during shifts as necessary to look professional and avoid carrying odors.
- Smile and maintain an even, friendly demeanor while on the job.
- Perform job tasks efficiently without rushing.
- Promote a positive attitude among staff.
- Handle stress and pressure with poise and tact.
- Be willing and available to stay late or through breaks, when needed, to assist with emergency or critical-care patients.
- Show respect for clients, team members, and animals (alive or deceased) at all times.
- Have the physical strength and ability to stand for an entire shift when needed, and be able to lift pets and objects weighing up to 50 pounds without assistance. Assist in lifting patients weighing more than 50 pounds.
- Maintain a list of tasks and engage in productive work during slow periods.
- Schedule technical and kennel staff.
- Supervise and direct technical and kennel staff.
- Direct on-the-job training of technical and kennel staff.
- Assist other employees as needed. Avoid waiting for coworkers to ask for assistance.
- Maintain your personal veterinary technician certificate, license, or registration.
- Assist in hiring new employees by advising candidates of openings, offering them applications, working with them to help evaluate their personalities and skill levels, and providing your opinion to the hiring manager.
- Participate in your performance appraisal, and, as requested, in those of others.
- Participate in all staff and training meetings.

- Keep up with new developments in the field by reading journals and attending continuing education. Attend off-site CE as required by the practice manager or as required to maintain your license.
- Organize and present training seminars for other support staff.
- Maintain constant vigilance regarding open doorways that could allow pets to escape from the facility.
- Maintain strict confidentiality regarding clients and patients for whom the practice provides veterinary services.
- Be prepared to handle any pet or facility emergency that may arise, including dog or cat fights, choking or strangulating animals, and facility fire or weather-related emergencies. Follow contingency plans.
- Follow established facility closing procedures to ensure the security of patients, staff, data, revenue, inventory, and the building.

Front-Office Tasks

- Know phone functions, including hold, intercom, transfer, forward, and three-way calling.
- Answer the phone by the third ring when receptionists are preoccupied or unavailable.
- Use patients' names during phone conversations with clients about their pets. Know each patient's sex so the pet can be called "he" or "she."
- Possess sufficient knowledge of animal husbandry and basic medicine to answer routine questions or refer calls to appropriate colleagues.

Client-Interaction Tasks

Patient-Admittance Tasks
- Cordially greet incoming clients and their pets, addressing each by name, and check them in when receptionists are busy.
- Admit patients to the hospital. Provide counseling and compassion for clients, answer their questions unless it is clear that the attending doctor should do so, and ensure that all admittance paperwork is properly completed.

- Complete and discuss financial estimates for clients as directed by doctors or the office manager.
- Provide clients with handouts and brochures regarding relevant medical conditions, surgeries, immunizations, internal and external parasites, pet health insurance, and diets.
- Assist clients with unruly or unrestrained pets.
- Transfer incoming patients to appropriate wards and ensure their comfort. Identify patients with cage cards and neck bands. Check for the presence of appropriate paperwork.

Pet-Identification Tasks

- Scan new patients and strays for microchips, tags, and tattoos. Identify and record microchip numbers, tattoos, and/or patient markings in patient records.
- Communicate with clients about the various pet-identification systems available, including tags, tattoos, and microchips.
- Assist clients in registering pet-identification information in the practice's computer system and in the appropriate national database.

Procedural Tasks

- As patients are admitted, build a surgery, procedure, and/or treatment schedule for the approval of the attending doctors.
- Develop each day's hospital census and/or client-update forms, starting with in-hospital patients, and assist with development of these forms as patients are admitted for day-procedures, surgeries, or hospitalization. Deliver copies to the front desk at established times.

Patient-Discharge Tasks

- Coordinate patient transfers with front-desk, kennel, and/or veterinarians.
- Prepare medications and prescriptions for dispensing as directed by the doctor. Ensure that each prescription label contains the following information: doctor's name; practice's name, address, and phone number including area code; date; patient's and client's name; medication name, strength and volume (or number); administration instructions including route of administration, such as by mouth or in the ear; and product's expiration date.

- Dispense medications. Discuss administration or application and potential side effects with owners as directed by doctors.
- Accurately invoice clients from charges on travel or circle sheets or records. Activate computer reminders and insert computerized notes, treatments, diagnostics, and diagnoses.
- Receive and record client payments.
- Discharge patients. Instruct clients on the care of patients at home, the timing of recheck appointments, and warnings of adverse effects of surgeries or medications.
- Assist grieving clients and comfort them. Be familiar with the grieving process. Always be sensitive to background chatter or conversations that could exacerbate the anxieties and grief clients experience during euthanasias or deaths of their pets.
- Provide clients with memorials of their dead-on-arrival, died-during-hospitalization, or euthanized pets, (e.g., locks of hair, paw prints, or paw molds). Return collars, leashes, and other accessories.
- Handle angry or grieving clients with a calm and reassuring manner. Be familiar with the grieving process. Always be sensitive to background chatter or conversations that could exacerbate the anxieties and grief clients experience during euthanasias or deaths of their pets.
- Assist clients to their vehicles if needed.

Medical-Record Management Tasks

- Understand the medical-record filing system.
- Locate medical files for hospitalized, surgical, or incoming patients.
- Record doctors' and technicians' notes in patients' computer records or on paper records.
- Make notes in patient files of all relevant phone or in-person conversations with clients, especially when notifying them of lab results. Place your initials after the entries.
- Verify and/or witness clients' statements regarding procedures, including euthanasias.
- Check files for completeness of notes, charges, callbacks, and reminders, making entries as needed.
- Accurately file all paper medical records.

Exam-Room Tasks

- Possess sufficient strength and assertiveness to effectively restrain patients and ensure the safety of clients and personnel.
- Clean and straighten exam rooms to prepare for incoming patients. Spray disinfectant on exam tables, wipe them clean, and dry them. Remove sources of offensive odors; empty trash if necessary. Check floors, walls, doors, and counters, and sweep or clean them as needed to remove hair, body fluids, and dirt.
- Obtain and record patient histories from clients.
- Answer questions and educate clients about basic pet care and procedures including nutrition; internal and external parasite control; immunization protocols; the administration of topical, oral, otic, and ophthalmic medications; spay and neuter procedures; and behavior and obedience training.
- Complete cursory overall examinations of patients and record your findings in the medical records.
- Identify external parasites.
- Perform suture removals, nail trims, and wing trims.
- Draw up vaccines and/or injections for administration.
- Vaccinate pets. Follow manufacturers' directions as well as AAFP guidelines for placement of injectable vaccines at appropriate sites.
- Dispose of used needles and syringes and other sharp objects as set forth by the practice's policy and OSHA standards.
- Keep a small notebook or personal digital assistant (PDA) in your pocket to record accurate instructions, particularly regarding the preparation and administering medications to be dispensed.
- Inform the practice manager or doctors immediately of all bite or scratch wounds you suffer so that reports can be made and you can be referred for timely medical care by a physician if necessary. Clean all wounds quickly and thoroughly.

Nursing-Care Tasks

Basic and Environmental Tasks
- Prioritize tasks to maximize clients' satisfaction and patients' health.

- Track comfort items that clients brought for hospitalized patients.
- Wash, dry, and store patients' bedding and the practice's towels. Bedding should be in good repair.
- Provide occupants with clean, soft bedding.
- Clean cages when they are soiled, and scoop or change litter boxes as needed.
- Maximize patients' comfort with a gentle and reassuring manner. Understand that actions that would constitute animal cruelty under state or local laws or the practice's policies will be grounds for immediate reprimand and/or termination.
- Monitor patients for vomit, blood, urine, and feces in the cage, and clean patients and cages as needed. Note unexpected incidents on cage cards or charts.
- Monitor patients' behaviors and note potentially aggressive behaviors. Use caution when handling aggressive or potentially aggressive pets. Request assistance when needed.
- Monitor changes in patients' conditions. Alert doctors to significant changes.
- Alert doctors to notable pathology identified during patients' exams.
- Follow isolation procedures. Prevent contact between contagious animals and others. Using the designated products and dilutions for disinfectants, properly disinfect your shoes, hands, and clothing before leaving isolation areas.
- Walk dogs on a double leash or on a leash within a fenced exercise area. Ensure that they are restrained and under your control at all times.
- Accurately assess patients' temperatures, pulse rates, and respiratory rates.
- Clip hair in a manner that minimizes clipper burn. Maintain, clean, and lubricate clipper blades on a regular basis.
- Complete and update cage cards.
- Use warning stickers and notations on cage cards and records as appropriate.
- Prior to discharge, remove patients' catheters and clean patients so that no body fluids or excrement are present.

Patient-Treatment Tasks
- Understand the mechanics and application of standards of asepsis.

- Properly calculate medication dosages and volumes of liquids or tablets to be administered to patients.
- Maintain IV catheters so fluids flow freely; flush and clean as needed.
- Monitor and maintain urinary-collection bags. Record urine production on charts.
- Administer IV, IM, SQ, and oral medications.
- Provide IV and SQ fluid therapy to patients. Maintain aseptic conditions. Understand the different types of fluids and additives used in the practice. Calculate, add, and administer medications through fluids. Calculate and administer proper fluid flow rates to patients.
- Monitor, adjust, and maintain IV infusion pumps.
- Administer routine enemas.
- Apply wound dressings and treatments. Maintain a clean site. Understand the applications for wet, dry, and wet-to-dry dressings.
- Apply bandages in a manner that ensures that the bandage protects and/or limits mobility and remains properly applied. Cover and maintain bandages as needed to preserve function and cleanliness.
- Use cotton swabs to clean ears, bulb syringes to flush them, curettes to remove debris, and catheters to irrigate ear canals. Administer ear treatments without causing trauma, and teach clients how to complete this task.
- Trim nails to the quick without causing bleeding.
- Provide physical therapy and hydrotherapy to patients as instructed.
- Provide medical grooming, including medicated baths, dips, and mat removal.
- Understand how to stop bleeding by using styptic pencils, powder or other means.
- Deflea patients with flea combs, flea sprays, spot-on topicals, baths, dips, or appropriate medication.
- Detick patients with tick-removal instruments or medications.
- Identify a patient's level of pain and possible causes of pain, and understand the medications and methods used to control pain.
- Assist kennel staff in medicating and treating boarders.

Technical Tasks

General Technical Tasks

- Restrain pets in a manner that allows necessary work to be performed, minimizes patient stress, and ensures their safety and that of other people.
- Safely and effectively apply and use restraint devices, including muzzles, towels, gloves, and cat bags.
- Perform venipunctures using patients' cephalic, saphenous, and jugular veins in a manner that minimizes trauma to patients and injury to veins and allows you to successfully obtain non-hemolyzed blood samples.
- Collect urine and fecal samples. Use fecal loops for stool collection as needed. When required, perform urinary catheterizations on male dogs or cystocenteses on male and female dogs, cats, and pocket pets.
- Aseptically place cephalic, saphenous, and jugular intravenous catheters without causing patient trauma.
- Perform needle aspirates and stain them as requested.
- Draw blood for transfusions. Type-match blood samples. Perform blood transfusions: set up filters for whole-blood administration, oversee administration of blood and blood products, and monitor patients for transfusion reactions.
- Set up and record diagnostic multi-lead ECG tracings.
- Collect and properly store canine semen.
- Make effective smears from vaginal swabs.
- Obtain ear swabs and cultures for analysis.
- Express anal sacs.
- Properly implant microchips and test their functionality.
- Neatly and accurately tattoo patients.
- Assist with euthanasia procedures. Hold off veins and release pressure at appropriate times when catheters are not used.

Emergency-Care Tasks

- Provide basic life support, including CPR, airway maintenance, and oxygen therapy.

- Apply temporary bandages or splints.
- Know where to find the emergency drug kit. Make sure products have not expired, and understand the basic uses for these drugs.
- Control bleeding using pressure bandages and tourniquets.
- Provide fluid and pharmacologic therapy under veterinary supervision.
- Provide cooling baths and/or enemas for heatstroke patients.

Laboratory Tasks
- Understand the paperwork and procedures of outside laboratories used by the practice.
- Maintain all laboratory test kits and reagents under proper environmental conditions.
- Maintain centrifuges, microscopes, and chemistry analyzers.
- Make slides of body fluids. Air-dry and stain them as directed.
- Make blood smears with properly feathered edges to ensure accurate interpretation.
- Evaluate blood smears to accurately assess platelet numbers, red and white cell morphology, and differential white counts. Recognize blood pathogens.
- Maintain stains and other supplies to ensure the best results. Prevent contamination of stains and replace them when ineffective or contaminated.
- Use proper stain techniques to maximize the diagnostic capability of prepared slides.
- Evaluate vaginal smears to determine stages of estrus.
- Evaluate fresh semen for evidence of fertility and sperm quality.
- Perform urinalyses. Properly use and record data from urine dipsticks. Measure specific gravity. Evaluate urine sediments for crystals, cells, and other material.
- Perform fecal examinations, including direct and flotation procedures.
- Perform and evaluate skin scrapings and ear smears.
- Complete routine ELISA tests, such as heartworm and feline viral tests.
- Perform CBCs and differentials.
- Set up, centrifuge, and read hematocrits.

- Use refractometers or chemistry analyzers to evaluate total protein levels of serum or other fluids.
- Set up and read Azostix® and blood glucose test strips.
- Use handheld glucometers to measure blood glucose values.
- Collect and prepare samples for bacterial and fungal cultures. Evaluate in-house cultures.
- Evaluate bleeding/clotting times.
- Maintain quality control by running control samples and periodically testing in-house results against results from an outside laboratory.

Surgical Tasks

- Develop or locate and maintain equipment and instrument maintenance logs.
- Serve as laser safety officer. Ensure the eye safety of veterinarians and staff present during laser surgery.
- Understand aseptic principles and apply them to surgical patients, instruments, equipment, and rooms.
- Know the names of instruments and where they are stored.
- Prepare the surgery suite(s) for incoming patients.
- Prepare patients for surgery. Clip surgical fields with straight margins. Minimize tissue trauma. Properly scrub and prepare surgical fields. Maintain clean fields when moving patients.
- Properly position and align patients for surgery.
- Use circulating warm-water baths and/or hot water bottles to maintain the body temperatures of anesthetic and surgical patients.
- Ground patients when using electrocautery.
- Properly scrub hands and arms for surgical cleanliness, and aseptically gown and glove yourself when called to assist or "scrub in."
- Assist surgeons with aseptic gowning and gloving.
- Anticipate surgeons' needs for assistance, instruments, and patient monitoring, and treatments.
- Monitor patients' recoveries. Protect patients from aspiration and hypothermia. Deflate cuffs and remove endotracheal tubes as soon as gag reflexes return.
- Stimulate and care for puppies and kittens removed by cesarean section.

- Maintain surgery logs with patients' names, doctors' names, procedures performed, types and amounts of preanesthetic and anesthetic agents, and surgical times.
- Maintain controlled-substance logs with patients' names, doctors' names, types and amounts of drugs used, amounts of drugs remaining, and your signature.
- Maintain logs of the number of hours surgical lasers are in use.
- Keep controlled drugs secured to meet Drug Enforcement Agency and state board specifications.
- Update patient records with drugs administered, procedures performed, and patient status during surgeries and recoveries.

Surgical Cleaning Tasks

- Clean operating rooms and equipment after use.
- Clean surgical prep and recovery areas.
- Wash, sterilize, and store endotracheal tubes.
- Dispose of used needles and syringes and other sharp objects as set forth by the practice's policy and OSHA standards.
- Clean surgical instruments by hand and/or ultrasonic cleaner.
- Operate and maintain the autoclave.
- Pack and autoclave instruments. Using lists of instruments or photos as guides, ensure that packs contain the proper numbers and types of instruments and that they are labeled with dates and types of packs. Apply pressure and temperature sterilization tape and/or monitors, and verify effectiveness after autoclaving.

Dental Tasks

- Know the names of surgical and dental instruments and their storage locations.
- Understand and use proper attire when operating dental equipment, including masks, eye protection, caps, and protective apparel such as a gown or scrubs.
- Recognize significant dental and gum disease, record it in patient records, and bring it to the attention of doctors.
- Perform dental scaling and polishing procedures without traumatizing the gingiva.
- Perform fluoride treatments.

- Perform dental extractions under the direction of attending doctors. Ensure full root removals or report incomplete extractions.
- Maintain proper dental records for each patient.

ANESTHETIC TASKS

- Be sufficiently familiar with the anesthetic machines to operate, maintain, and repair them.
- Routinely check and change soda lime. Record dates of soda-lime changes on the machines.
- Check anesthetic hoses for leaks and internal contaminants.
- Ensure that the anesthetic scavenging system is functional.
- Understand the differences between closed- and open-circuit administration of anesthetic agents, adjustments needed for oxygen flow rates, and anesthetic percentages used for each.
- Regularly check the level of inhalant anesthetic in vaporizers. Add anesthetic as needed.
- Check pressures in oxygen tanks regularly and replace tanks at appropriate times. Check regularly for leaks in oxygen hoses and couplings.
- Connect oxygen tanks to anesthetic machines without damaging gaskets. Maintain spare gaskets and replace them if they are damaged.
- Test endotracheal tube cuffs for leaks prior to use and replace them.
- Know the volume of air that should be used to inflate various-sized cuffs to pressure levels that prevent leakage without traumatizing tracheas.
- Generally understand the various anesthetic agents used for different patients.
- Administer preanesthetic drugs to surgical patients as directed. Record times of administration.
- Preoxygenate surgical patients that are at particular risk for oxygen deprivation as directed.
- Administer IV, IM, and inhalation anesthetic agents safely.
- Estimate endotracheal tube diameters for patients. Safely pass endotracheal tubes and ensure proper fits.
- Use a laryngoscope or other light source as needed to pass tubes.
- Check patients for proper respiratory function during intubation to ensure that tubes are in the trachea and not the esophagus.

- Monitor surgical patients by tracking anesthetic depths, heart rates, respiratory rates, temperatures, pulse oximetry, and ECGs during anesthetic procedures.
- Adjust gas anesthesia for each patient to safely maintain proper surgical planes. Administer additional injectable anesthetics within safety guidelines as needed to maintain desired surgical depths.
- Use palpebral, toe pinch, and corneal reflexes to assess and maintain necessary surgical planes.
- Maintain anesthetic log books so as to be in compliance with AAHA and state board standards.

Imaging Tasks

Radiology Tasks

- Maintain radiographic, developing, and shielding equipment to maximize patients' and employees' safety. Record maintenance data.
- Know how to perform radiographic contrast studies, such as barium swallows, upper and lower contrast studies of the GI system, excretory urograms, and cystourethrograms.
- Minimize radiation hazards. Use protective equipment and wear exposure badges during radiographic exposures.
- Properly measure patients for effective translation to radiograph machine settings.
- Develop, use, adjust, and maintain a radiograph technique chart that minimizes waste caused by erroneous exposures.
- Position patients to obtain diagnostic-quality radiographs of skeletal anatomy, internal organs, superficial lesions, or extremities.
- Consistently use right and left markers.
- Adjust machine settings to correct technique failures.
- Properly store radiograph cassettes and unexposed film.
- Understand darkroom procedures, including film labeling, film developing, and plate refilling. Ensure that labels contain dates

and the practice's, clients', and patients' names, and that these are impregnated on the radiograph film as required by state boards or standards of veterinary practice. Develop film with an automatic processor or hand process with tanks.

- Change the developer and fixer in tanks at appropriate times.
- Understand the radiograph filing system. Properly label and file films.
- Maintain a radiograph log book that complies with AAHA standards and/or state laws.

Ultrasound and Endoscopy Tasks

- Prepare patients for ultrasound.
- Warm the ultrasound gel before use.
- Properly restrain and position patients for ultrasonography.
- Perform introductory ultrasound surveys as directed.
- Clean and maintain ultrasound equipment.
- Properly clean, handle, maintain, and store all endoscopic equipment.

Inventory-Management Tasks

- Discuss new products with detail representatives and doctors.
- Develop and maintain contacts for detail reps and sources of drugs and supplies.
- Maintain lists of medications, vaccines, pet food, and/or hospital supplies to determine levels of inventory on hand. Place orders for additional supplies on demand, if so instructed, or report items needed to the ordering manager.
- Receive and stock supplies, matching invoices with packaged goods. Report all shortages, overages, and damaged goods.
- Ensure that medical supplies are always available.
- Regularly check for outdated supplies. Remove and replace them as instructed by the practice manager.

CHAPTER 7

VETERINARY TECHNICIAN TRAINING SCHEDULE

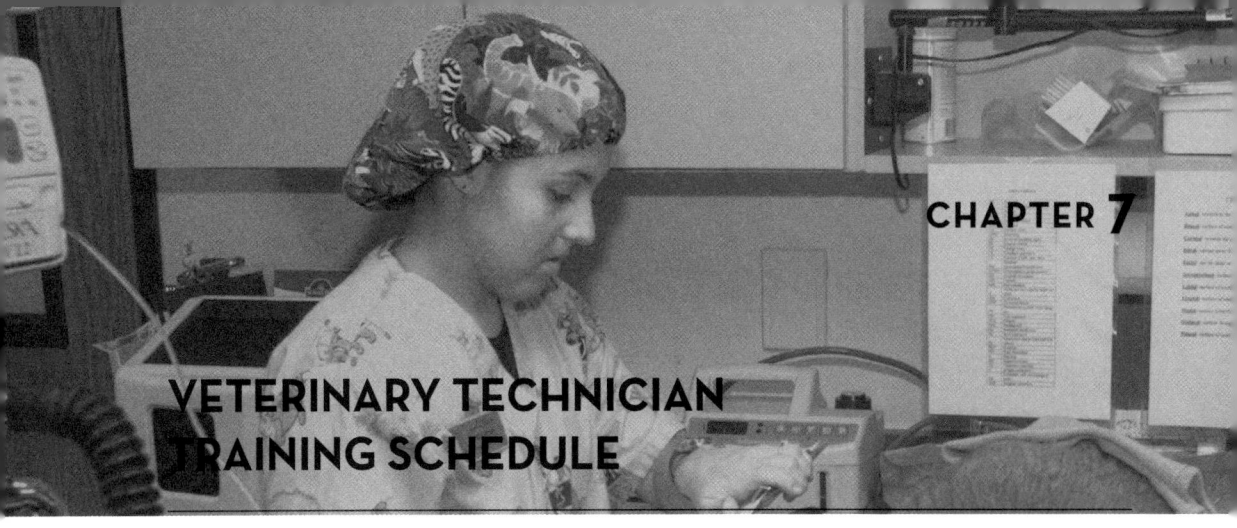

Veterinary technicians have varying degrees of knowledge, education, training, and experience. Some technicians are fresh out of AVMA-accredited schools, while others acquired their skills on the job. Some have passed the national veterinary technician examination (VTNE) and state certification or registration exams. Others have not completed state testing or certification requirements.

Because there is such a wide variation in the skill levels of newly hired veterinary technicians, developing standardized training schedules for them is a challenge. We recommend that managers follow the subsequent guidelines to develop individualized training schedules for each newly hired technician, in addition to using the guidelines offered in Chapter 1.

1. Print a hard copy of the technician training schedule for each newly hired technician. If you will be modifying the schedule electronically, we recommend using your word processing software's "save as" function to save the new version and preserve the content of the original "master schedule." As suggested in Chapter 1, this can be done using a series of folders (e.g., C: //Employees/job descriptions/veterinary techs/Sally Brown's JD 11-1-05). We recommend naming each new document with the new employee's name, followed by the most current date.

2. Evaluate the first section in the following training schedule, entitled "At the time of hire, new technicians should already be able to." Review each task in this section with newly hired technicians to assess whether they already possess the knowledge and skill required to complete the task. If they are truly competent in a task, cross it off the hard copy or delete it from the electronic version. Continue in this manner until all tasks in this section have been considered.

3. The tasks remaining are those that the new staff person needs to learn. Establish a training schedule for these remaining tasks that fits the desired learning curve. The initial list contains the authors' suggested time frames for learning these tasks. They include: within the first week (1w), first month (1m), first three

months (3m), and first six months (6m), and after the first six months (6+m).

Cut and paste the remaining tasks in the electronic version of this document to the appropriate time periods appearing later in the training schedule. For example, if the newly hired technician must learn to apply wound dressings and treatments, that task could be moved to the "By the end of month six, new technicians should have learned to," section.

4. The final copy of the customized training document should be identified with the employee's name and date and saved to floppy disk or hard drive. Hard copies should be printed for easy reference by the new veterinary technicians, trainers, and managers.

At the time of hire, if new technicians or nurses are not already familiar with or capable of performing the following tasks, they should be able to do so within the timelines noted below:

General Knowledge and Tasks

- Be reasonably familiar with breeds and coat colors. (3m)
- Know and use standard medical and business abbreviations. (1m)
- Use proper medical terminology when speaking and writing, simplifying it for clients who have a limited understanding of medicine. (3m)
- Be familiar with infectious diseases, including their prevention and steps to reduce or eliminate transmission. Know the most common zoonotic diseases (infections from animal to humans). (3m)

Front-Office Tasks

- Possess sufficient knowledge of animal husbandry and basic medicine to answer routine questions or refer calls to appropriate colleagues. (6+m)

Client-Interaction Tasks

- Communicate with clients about the various pet-identification systems available, including tags, tattoos, and microchips. (1m)
- Scan new patients and strays for microchips, tags, and tattoos.

Identify and record microchip numbers, tattoos, and/or patient markings in patient records. (1m)

- Prepare medications and prescriptions for dispensing as directed by the doctor. Ensure that each prescription label contains the following information: doctor's name; practice's name, address, and phone number including area code; date; patient's and client's name; medication name, strength and volume (or number); administration instructions including route of administration, such as by mouth or in the ear; and product's expiration date. (3m)
- Be familiar with the grieving process. (3m)

Exam-Room Tasks

- Obtain and record patient histories from clients. (3m)
- Complete cursory overall examinations of patients and record your findings in medical records. (6+m)
- Identify external parasites visually or with the aid of a microscope. (1m)
- Perform suture removals, nail trims, and wing trims. (1m)
- Draw up vaccines and/or injections for administration. (1m)
- Vaccinate pets. Follow manufacturers' directions as well as AAFP guidelines for placement of injectable vaccines at appropriate sites. (1m)

Nursing-Care Tasks

- Monitor changes in patients' conditions. Alert doctors to significant changes. (1m)
- Accurately assess patients' temperatures, pulse rates, and respiratory rates. (1w)
- Clip hair in a manner that minimizes clipper burns. Maintain, clean, and lubricate clipper blades on a regular basis. (1m)
- Properly calculate medication dosages and volumes of liquids or tablets to be administered to patients. (6m)
- Maintain IV catheters so fluids flow freely; flush and clean as needed. (1m)
- Monitor and maintain urinary collection bags. Record urine production on charts. (1w)

- Administer IV, IM, SQ, and oral medications. (1m)
- Provide IV and SQ fluid therapy to patients. Maintain aseptic conditions. Understand the different types of fluids and additives used. Calculate, add, and administer medications through fluids. Calculate and administer proper fluid flow rates to patients. (6m)
- Monitor, adjust, and maintain IV infusion pumps. (1m)
- Administer routine enemas. (3m)
- Apply wound dressings and treatments. Maintain a clean site. Understand the applications for wet, dry, and wet-to-dry dressings. (6m)
- Apply bandages in a manner that ensures that the bandage protects and/or limits mobility and remains properly applied. Cover and maintain bandages as needed to preserve function and cleanliness. (6m)
- Use cotton swabs to clean ears, bulb syringes to flush them, curettes to remove debris, and catheters to irrigate ear canals. Administer ear treatments without causing trauma, and teach clients how to complete this task. (6m)
- Trim nails to the quick without causing bleeding. (1w)
- Understand how to stop bleeding by using styptic pencils, powder, or other means. (1m)
- Provide physical therapy and hydrotherapy to patients as instructed. (6m)
- Provide medical grooming, including medicated baths, dips, nail trims, and mat removal. (1m)
- Deflea patients with flea combs, flea sprays, spot-on topicals, baths, dips, or appropriate medication. (1w)
- Detick patients with tick-removal instruments or medications. (1w)
- Identify a patient's level of pain and possible causes of pain, and understand the medications and methods used to control pain. (3m)
- Assist kennel staff in medicating and treating boarders. (1m)
- Understand the mechanics and application of standards of asepsis. (6m)

Technical Tasks

Note that we've left the subcategories of tasks (e.g., general technical, emergency-care) under this category so that they may broken up into manageable chunks.

General Technical Tasks

- Restrain pets in a manner that allows necessary work to be performed, minimizes patient stress, and ensures their safety and that of other people. Safely and effectively apply and use restraint devices, including muzzles, towels, gloves, and cat bags. (1m)
- Safely and effectively apply and use restraint devices, including muzzles, towels, gloves, and cat bags. (1m)
- Perform venipunctures using patients' cephalic, saphenous, and jugular veins in a manner that minimizes trauma to patients and injury to veins and allows you to successfully obtain non-hemolyzed blood samples. (3m)
- Collect urine and fecal samples. Use fecal loops for stool collection as needed. When required, perform urinary catheterizations on male dogs or cystocenteses on male and female dogs, cats, and pocket pets. (6+m)
- Aseptically place cephalic, saphenous, and jugular intravenous catheters without causing significant patient trauma. (6m)
- Perform needle aspirates and stain them as requested. (6+m)
- Draw blood for transfusions. Type-match blood samples. Perform blood transfusions: set up filters for whole-blood administration, oversee administration of blood and blood products, and monitor patients for transfusion reactions. (6+m)
- Set up and record diagnostic multi-lead ECG tracings. (6m)
- Collect and properly store canine semen. (6+m)
- Make effective smears from vaginal swabs. (6m)
- Obtain ear swabs for cytology and cultures. (3m)
- Express anal sacs. (3m)
- Properly implant microchips and test their functionality. (1m)
- Neatly and accurately tattoo patients. (3m)
- Assist with euthanasia procedures. Hold off veins and release pressure at appropriate times when catheters are not used. (1m)

Emergency-Care Tasks

- Provide basic life support, including CPR, airway maintenance, and oxygen therapy. (3m)
- Apply temporary bandages or splints. (6m)
- Control bleeding using pressure bandages and tourniquets. (3m)
- Provide fluid and pharmacologic therapy under veterinary supervision. (1m)

- Provide cooling baths and/or enemas for heatstroke patients. (1m)

Laboratory Tasks

- Maintain all laboratory test kits and reagents under proper environmental conditions. (1w)
- Maintain centrifuges, microscopes, and chemistry analyzers. (3m)
- Make slides of body fluids. Air-dry and stain them as directed. (3m)
- Make blood smears with properly feathered edges to ensure accurate interpretation. (3m)
- Evaluate blood smears to accurately assess platelet numbers, red- and white-cell morphology, and differential white counts. Recognize blood pathogens. (6m)
- Maintain stains and other supplies to ensure the best results. (1m)
- Use proper stain techniques to maximize the diagnostic capability of prepared slides. (3m)
- Evaluate vaginal smears to determine stages of estrus. (6m)
- Evaluate fresh semen for evidence of fertility and sperm quality. (6m)
- Perform urinalyses. Properly use and record data from urine dipsticks. Measure specific gravity. Evaluate urine sediments for crystals, cells, and other material. (6m)
- Perform fecal examinations, including direct and flotation procedures. (1m)
- Perform and evaluate skin scrapings and ear smears. (6m)
- Complete routine ELISA tests, such as heartworm and feline viral tests. (1m)
- Perform CBCs and differentials. (6m)
- Set up, centrifuge, and read hematocrits. (1m)
- Use refractometers or chemistry analyzers to evaluate total protein levels of serum or other fluids. (1m)
- Set up and read Azostix® and blood glucose strip tests. (1m)
- Use handheld glucometers to measure blood glucose values. (1m)
- Collect and prepare samples for bacterial and fungal cultures. Evaluate in-house cultures. (6m)
- Evaluate bleeding/clotting times. (6m)

- Maintain quality controls by running control samples and periodically testing in-house results against results from an outside laboratory. (1m)

Surgical Tasks

- Understand aseptic principles and apply them to surgical patients, instruments, equipment, and rooms. (6m)
- Prepare patients for surgery. Clip surgical fields with straight margins. Minimize tissue trauma. Properly scrub and prepare surgical fields. Maintain clean fields when moving patients. (1m)
- Properly position and align patients for surgery. (1m)
- Properly scrub hands and arms for surgical cleanliness, and aseptically gown and glove when called to assist or "scrub in." (1m)
- Assist surgeons with aseptic gowning and gloving. (1m)
- Monitor patients' anesthetic recoveries. Protect patients from aspiration and hypothermia. Deflate cuffs and remove patients' endotracheal tubes as soon as gag reflexes return. (3m)
- Stimulate and care for puppies and kittens removed by cesarean section. (3m)

Surgical Cleaning Tasks

- Clean operating rooms and equipment after use. (1m)
- Clean surgical prep and recovery areas. (1m)
- Wash, sterilize, and store endotracheal tubes using techniques that prevent the spread of disease. (1m)
- Clean surgical instruments. Operate ultrasonic instrument cleaner. Repack and sterilize instruments. Use lists and/or photos with labels to ensure that packs contain the proper number and type of instruments. Label the packs with the date and type of pack. Apply pressure and temperature indicators, and verify changes after autoclaving. (1m)
- Operate and maintain the autoclave. (1m)

Dental Tasks

- Recognize significant dental and gum disease, record it in patient records, and bring it to the attention of doctors. (3m)
- Perform dental scaling and polishing procedures without traumatizing the gingiva. (3m)
- Perform fluoride treatments. (3m)

- Perform dental extractions under the direction of attending doctors. Ensure full root removals or report incomplete extractions. (6m)
- Maintain proper dental records for each patient. (6m)

ANESTHETIC TASKS

- Routinely check and change soda lime. Record dates of soda-lime changes on machines. (1m)
- Check anesthetic hoses for leaks and internal contaminants. (1m)
- Ensure that the anesthetic scavenging system is functional. (1m)
- Understand the differences between the closed- and open-circuit administration of anesthetic agents, adjustments needed for oxygen flow rates, and anesthetic percentages used for each. (6m)
- Regularly check the level of inhalant anesthetic in vaporizers. Add anesthetic as needed. (1m)
- Check pressures in oxygen tanks regularly and replace tanks at appropriate times. Check regularly for leaks in oxygen hoses and couplings. (1m)
- Connect oxygen tanks to anesthetic machines without damaging gaskets. Maintain spare gaskets and replace them if they are damaged. (1m)
- Test endotracheal tube cuffs for leaks prior to use, and replace them. (1m)
- Know the volume of air that should be used to inflate various-sized cuffs to pressure levels that prevent leakage without traumatizing tracheas. (6m)
- Generally understand the various anesthetic agents used for different patients. (6m)
- Administer preanesthetic drugs to surgical patients as directed. Record times of administration. (1m)
- Preoxygenate surgical patients that are at particular risk for oxygen deprivation as directed. (1m)
- Administer IV, IM, and inhalation anesthetic agents safely. (6m)
- Estimate endotracheal tube diameters for patients. Safely and efficiently pass endotracheal tubes and ensure proper fits. (6m)
- Use a laryngoscope or other light source as needed to pass tubes. (6m)

- Check patients for proper respiratory function during intubation to ensure that tubes are in the trachea and not in the esophagus. (6m)
- Monitor surgical patients by tracking anesthetic depths, heart rates, respiratory rates, temperatures, pulse oximetry, and ECGs during anesthetic procedures. (3m)
- Adjust gas anesthesia for each patient to safely maintain proper surgical planes. Administer additional injectable anesthetics within safety guidelines as needed to maintain desired surgical depths. (6m)
- Use palpebral, toe pinch, and corneal reflexes to assess and maintain necessary surgical planes. (3m)

Imaging Tasks

- Know how to perform radiographic contrast studies, such as barium swallows, upper and lower contrast studies of the GI system, excretory urograms, and cystourethrograms. (6+m)
- Minimize radiation hazards. Use protective equipment and wear exposure badges during radiographic exposures. (1w)
- Properly measure patients for effective application of radiograph machine settings. (1m)
- Develop, use, adjust, and maintain a radiograph technique chart that minimizes waste caused by erroneous exposures. (6m)
- Position patients to obtain diagnostic-quality radiographs of skeletal anatomy, internal organs, superficial lesions, or extremities. (3m)
- Adjust machine settings to correct technique failures. (6m)
- Properly store radiograph cassettes and unexposed film. (1m)
- Understand darkroom procedures, including film labeling, film developing, and plate refilling. Ensure that labels contain dates and the practice's, clients', and patients' names, and that these are impregnated in the radiograph film as required by state boards or standards of veterinary practice. Develop film with an automatic processor or hand process with tanks. (1m)
- Change the developer and fixer in tanks at appropriate times. (1m)
- Prepare patients for ultrasound. (1m)

- Properly restrain and position patients for ultrasonography. (1m)
- Clean and maintain ultrasound equipment. (1m)
- Properly clean, handle, maintain, and store all endoscopic equipment. (1m)

Week One

If there are tasks that a new technician should have already mastered at the time of hire (see pages 84–92), but hasn't, and should master by the end of week one, cut and paste them here. By the end of week one, new technicians should have learned to:

General Knowledge and Tasks

- Follow OSHA standards. Be able to find Material Safety Data Sheets quickly.
- Maintain accurate personal time cards.
- Participate in their performance appraisals, and, as requested, in those of others.

Front-Office Tasks

- Know phone functions, including hold, intercom, transfer, forward, and three-way calling.

Client-Interaction Tasks

- As patients are admitted, build a surgery, procedure, and/or treatment schedule for the approval of the attending doctor.
- Coordinate patient transfers with front desk, kennel, and/or veterinarians.

Medical-Record Management Tasks

- Understand the medical-record filing system.

- Locate medical files for hospitalized, surgical, or incoming patients.
- Accurately file all paper medical records. Know all possible locations for storage of records of hospitalized patients.

Exam-Room Tasks

- Clean and straighten exam rooms to prepare them for incoming patients.

Nursing-Care Tasks

- Track comfort items clients brought to the practice for hospitalized patients.
- Wash, dry, and store patients' bedding and the practice's towels. Bedding should be in good repair.
- Follow isolation procedures. Prevent contact between contagious animals and others. Using the designated products and dilutions for disinfectants, properly disinfect your shoes, hands, and clothing before leaving isolation areas.
- Complete and update cage cards.
- Use warning stickers and notations.

Technical Tasks

- Know where to find the emergency drug kit, make sure that products have not expired, and understand the basic uses for these drugs.
- Serve as laser safety officer. Ensure the eye safety of veterinarians and staff present during laser surgery.
- Prepare the surgery suite(s) for incoming patients.
- Maintain surgery logs with patients' names, doctors' names, procedures performed, types and amounts of preanesthetic and anesthetic agents, and surgical times.
- Maintain controlled-substance logs with patients' names, doctors' names, types and amounts of drugs used, amounts of drugs remaining, and your signature.

- Maintain logs of the number of hours surgical lasers are in use.
- Keep controlled drugs secured in a manner that meet Drug Enforcement Agency and state board specifications.
- Update patient records with drugs administered, procedures performed, and patient status during surgeries and recoveries.
- Dispose of used needles and syringes and other sharp objects as set forth by the practice's policy and according to OSHA standards.
- Maintain anesthetic log books so as to be in compliance with AAHA and state board standards.

Imaging Tasks

- Understand the radiograph filing system. Properly label and file films.
- Maintain a radiograph log book that complies with AAHA standards and/or state laws.

Month One

If there are tasks that a new technician should have already mastered at the time of hire (see pages 84–92), but hasn't, and should master by the end of month one, cut and paste them here. By the end of month one, new technicians should have learned to:

General Knowledge and Tasks

- Maintain a list of tasks and engage in productive work during slow periods.
- Follow established facility closing procedures to ensure the security of patients, staff, data, revenue, inventory, and the building.

Front-Office Tasks

- Answer the phone by the third ring when receptionists are preoccupied or unavailable.

CLIENT-INTERACTION TASKS

- Complete and discuss financial estimates for clients as directed by doctors or the office manager.
- Provide clients with handouts and brochures regarding relevant medical conditions, surgeries, immunizations, internal and external parasites, pet health insurance, and diets.
- Transfer incoming patients to appropriate wards and ensure their comfort. Identify patients with cage cards and neck bands. Check for the presence of appropriate paperwork.
- Develop each day's hospital census and/or client update forms, starting with in-hospital patients, and assist with development of these forms as patients are admitted for day-procedures, surgeries, or hospitalization. Deliver copies to the front desk at established times.
- Dispense medications. Discuss administration or application and potential side effects with owners as directed by doctors.
- Provide clients with memorials of their dead-on-arrival, died-during-hospitalization, or euthanized pets, (e.g., locks of hair, paw prints, or paw molds). Return collars, leashes, and other accessories.

MEDICAL-RECORD MANAGEMENT TASKS

- Record doctors' and technicians' notes in patients' computer records or on paper records.
- Make notes in patients' files of all relevant phone or in-person conversations with clients, especially when notifying them of lab results. Place your initials after entries.
- Check files for completeness of notes, charges, callbacks, and reminders, making entries as needed.

EXAM-ROOM TASKS

- Answer questions and educate clients about basic pet care and procedures, including nutrition; internal and external parasite control; immunization protocols; the administration of topical, oral, otic, and ophthalmic medications; spay and neuter procedures; and behavior and obedience training.

Technical Tasks

- Understand the paperwork and procedures of outside laboratories used by the practice.
- Develop or locate and maintain equipment and instrument maintenance logs.
- Know the names of surgical and dental instruments and their storage locations.
- Be sufficiently familiar with the anesthetic machines to operate, maintain, and repair them.
- Maintain radiographic, developing, and shielding equipment to maximize patients' and employees' safety. Record maintenance data.

Inventory-Management Tasks

- Receive and stock supplies, matching invoices with packaged goods. Report all shortages, overages, and damaged goods.

Month Three

If there are tasks that a new technician should have already mastered at the time of hire (see pages XX–XX), but hasn't, and should master by the end of month three, cut and paste them here. By the end of month three, new technicians should have learned to:

Month Six

If there are tasks that a new technician should have already mastered at the time of hire (see pages 84–92), but hasn't, and should master by the end of month six, cut and paste them here.

By the end of month six, new technicians should have learned to:

General Knowledge and Tasks

- Schedule technical and kennel staff.
- Assist in hiring new employees by advising candidates of openings, offering applications, working with them to help evaluate their personalities and skill levels, and providing your opinion to the hiring manager.
- Organize and present training seminars for other support staff.

Client-Interaction Tasks

- Cordially greet incoming clients and their pets, addressing each by name, and check them in when receptionists are busy.
- Admit patients to the hospital. Provide counseling and compassion for clients, answer their questions unless it is clear that the attending doctor should do so, and ensure that all admittance paperwork is properly completed.
- Assist clients in registering pet-identification information in the practice's computer system and in the appropriate national database.
- Accurately invoice clients from charges on travel or circle sheets or records. Activate computer reminders and insert computerized notes, treatments, diagnostics, and diagnoses.
- Receive and record client payments.
- Discharge patients. Instruct clients on the care of patients at home, the timing of recheck appointments, and warnings of adverse effects of surgeries or medications.

Inventory-Management Tasks

- Discuss new products with detail representatives and doctors, and gather sufficient information to present information about such items to the doctors and/or manager.
- Develop and maintain contacts for detail reps and sources of drugs and supplies.
- Maintain lists of medications, vaccines, pet food, and/or hospital supplies to determine the levels of inventory on hand. Place

orders for additional supplies on demand, if so instructed, or report items needed to the ordering manager.

Month Twelve

If there are tasks that a new technician should have already mastered at the time of hire (see pages 84–92), but hasn't, and should master by the end of month twelve, cut and paste them here. By the end of month twelve, new technicians should have learned to:

Imaging Tasks

- Perform introductory ultrasound surveys as directed.

CHAPTER 8

KENNEL ASSISTANT JOB DESCRIPTION

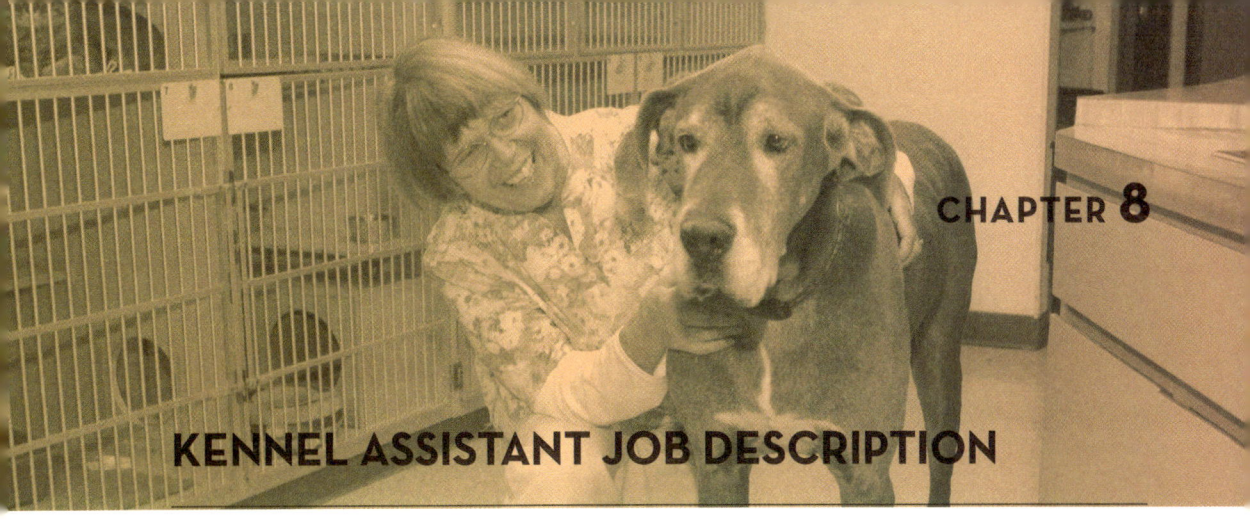

Veterinary kennel assistants (also called animal caretakers) are responsible for the day-to-day care of patients and boarders. This includes feeding, watering, cleaning, walking, bathing, and monitoring the well being of dogs, cats and, occasionally, other companion animals. Kennel assistants must have sufficient physical strength, mobility, and stamina to lift and/or move heavy pets and objects, the dexterity and confidence to administer medications, and the ability to monitor pets for signs of distress or disease. It is essential that they have the ability and willingness to learn and the desire to provide gentle, compassionate care for boarded and hospitalized pets. Kennel experience is not always a prerequisite for this position.

General Knowledge and Tasks

General Knowledge

- Know the range of services the practice provides and the species it treats.
- Be reasonably familiar with breeds and coat colors.
- Follow OSHA standards. Be able to find Material Safety Data Sheets quickly.
- Know and use standard medical and business abbreviations.
- Use proper medical terminology when speaking and writing.
- Be familiar with infectious diseases, including their prevention and steps to reduce or eliminate transmission. Know the most common zoonotic diseases.
- Competently speak and write the English language.
- Competently speak a second language commonly used at the practice.

General Tasks

- Always be in position and prepared to work by the start of each scheduled shift.

- Maintain accurate personal time cards.
- Maintain a professional appearance while at work, including clean and pressed uniforms or clothes. Change clothes daily as necessary to look professional and avoid carrying odors.
- Maintain an even, friendly demeanor while on the job. Perform job tasks efficiently without rushing.
- Smile and maintain an even, friendly demeanor while on the job.
- Handle stress and pressure with poise and tact.
- Show respect for clients, team members, and animals (alive or deceased) at all times.
- Have the physical strength and ability to stand for an entire shift when needed, and be able to lift pets and objects weighing up to 50 pounds without assistance, handle repetitive up-and-down or back-and-forth motions, and work while bending. Assist in lifting patients weighing more than 50 pounds.
- Maintain a list of tasks and engage in productive work during slow periods.
- Assist other employees as needed. Avoid waiting for coworkers to ask for assistance.
- Assist in hiring new employees by advising candidates of openings and working with the kennel or practice manager and the applicants to help evaluate their personalities and skill levels.
- Keep up with new developments in the field through journals and continuing education. Attend off-site continuing education as required by the practice manager.
- Participate in your performance appraisal, and, as requested, in those of others.
- Participate in all staff and training meetings.
- Be willing and able to teach other staff members kennel skills.
- Answer preliminary questions from interested parties regarding stray and adoptable animals.
- Conduct tours of the practice and/or kennel. Before each tour, ensure that the facility is orderly and that staff and patients are prepared for tours.
- Maintain constant vigilance regarding open doorways that could allow pets to escape from the facility.
- Maintain strict confidentiality regarding clients and patients for whom the practice provides veterinary services.

- Be prepared to handle any pet or facility emergency that may arise, including dog or cat fights, choking or strangulating animals, and facility fire or weather-related emergencies. Follow contingency plans.
- Follow established facility closing procedures to ensure the security of patients, boarders, and the building.

CLIENT-INTERACTION TASKS

PATIENT-ADMITTANCE TASKS

- Cordially greet incoming clients and patients, addressing each by name.
- Check on the immunization status of arriving pets before admitting them to the facility.
- Advise clients of recommended services, such as exercise/play time and grooming, for their pets and of special call-in times to check on patients or boarders.
- Explain special programs offered by the practice.
- Advise clients of significant changes in policies or services since their last visit.
- Obtain and record contact information from clients to ensure that they or their agents can be reached during pets' stays.
- Ensure that all boarding admission paperwork has been completed.
- Administer tick and/or flea repellants or pesticides at the time patients are admitted as directed by the kennel manager.
- Take custody of pets from clients. Restrain dogs with the practice's leashes. Label and store clients' collars and leashes and return them to clients promptly when pets are retrieved from the facility.
- Note special instructions given by clients.
- Assist clients with unruly or unrestrained pets. Ensure that all dogs are leashed and that cats and smaller pets are caged. Isolate aggressive pets. Request assistance as needed.
- Weigh pets and record weights when they are admitted.
- Walk or carry pets to the appropriate wards. Apply identification bands. Settle pets comfortably in their assigned cages and runs.

Provide fresh water, if permitted, and clean bedding. Mark cages and runs with pets' cage cards.
- Make sure that all kennel and cage doors are properly secured after admitting or moving patients and before leaving the facility at the end of a shift.

Patient-Discharge Tasks

- Provide clients with summary evaluations of their pets' boarding stays. Advise them of significant events during their pets' boarding, including changes in anxiety and/or signs of illness, such as constant barking (dogs) or hiding (cats), loss of appetite, diarrhea, excessive thirst, sneezing, or coughing.
- On the day of discharge, gather pets' toys, bedding, and food in preparation for discharge.
- Check all pets for cleanliness prior to discharge. Clean, bathe, and/or groom pets prior to discharge as needed. Assess additional fees as directed. Discharge pets.
- Measure and record pets' exit weights for comparison against entry weights.
- Handle angry or grieving clients with a calm, compassionate, and reassuring manner.
- Assist clients to their cars if needed.

Pet-Care Tasks

Examination and Restraint Tasks

- Restrain pets in a manner that allows necessary work to be performed, minimizes stress to pets, and ensures the safety of pets and people.
- Evaluate incoming animals for obvious signs of disease and readily felt skin or body tumors. Find and identify external parasites. Bring noted problems to the attention of pet owners and the support staff for discussion and resolution prior to admittance.
- Know and use, when appropriate, various techniques to restrain fractious pets, including:
  1. muzzles, choke collars, Gentle Leader" headcollars, body harnesses, collars, cat bags, and "rabies poles";

2. blankets, towels, or nets to trap and move cats, dogs, and pocket pets;
3. collars and lead ropes through cage doors or chain-link fences or over tables; and
4. use of physical restraint using your body, hands, and/or arms.

- Aid veterinarians and technicians in evaluating incoming animals through examinations and health tests. Assist in administering immunizations.
- Use warning stickers and notations on cage cards and records as appropriate.

Contagious-Disease Tasks

- Follow isolation procedures for contagious or potentially contagious animals. Using the designated products and dilutions for disinfectants, properly disinfect your shoes, hands, and clothing before leaving isolation areas.
- Follow the practice's procedures and state guidelines in handling suspected or potential rabies cases. Inform the kennel manager, veterinary technicians, or doctors of signs that patients are having difficulty swallowing, exhibiting rear- or front-leg weakness, or exhibiting other neurological abnormalities.

Pet-Care and Monitoring Tasks

- Wash, dry, and store patients' bedding and the practice's towels. Bedding should be in good repair. Wash surgical towels separately.
- Maximize pets' comfort with a gentle and reassuring manner. Understand that actions that would constitute animal cruelty under state or local laws or the practice's policies will be grounds for immediate reprimand and/or termination.
- Ensure birds and exotic pets' needs and environmental conditions are met, including proper housing, perches, bedding, and diet.
- When transferring boarders to new locations, provide them with clean, soft bedding and fresh water.
- Walk dogs on a double leash or on a leash within a fenced exercise area. Ensure that they are restrained and under your control at all times.
- Provide individual or group playtime for boarders at clients' request and as directed by the practice or kennel manager. Ensure pets' safety and well-being at all times.

- Prepare meals according to clients' instructions, and feed animals. Note the volume of food eaten or rejected on cage cards or kennel logs.
- Withhold food and water from pets scheduled for or recovering from surgical procedures and anesthesia as directed.
- Rinse and refill water pails and dishes at least once daily. Wash and disinfect them as needed during pets' stays.
- Monitor pets and kennels/cages for urine, feces, vomit, and blood. When noted, clean pets, runs, play areas, litter pans, and cages or runs immediately. Note incidents on cage cards or kennel logs.
- Collect and save urine and fecal samples as requested.
- Continuously monitor pets in your care. Pay particular attention to signs of distress, illness, or injury.
- Know the key symptoms of emergency medical problems likely to be exhibited by boarders. Immediately notify the kennel manager or veterinary staff members if you observe any of the following clinical signs:
    1. Dogs or cats that are unable to or are straining to urinate or defecate
    2. Dogs or cats in heat
    3. Dogs suffering from gastric dilatation and volvulus (GDV or bloat), (i.e., bloated abdomens, unproductive vomiting, vomiting thick ropy saliva, and/or general discomfort)
    4. Difficult, heavy, or rapid breathing
    5. Sneezing, coughing, or ocular discharges
    6. Listlessness
    7. Loss of balance
    8. Inability to rise
    9. Anxiety
    10. Seizures
    11. Significant vomiting and/or diarrhea, especially bloody or foul-smelling diarrhea
    12. Bleeding
- Monitor boarders' behaviors and note potentially aggressive behaviors. Use caution when handling aggressive or potentially aggressive pets. Request assistance when needed for personal safety or for the safety of other boarders.

- Identify a patient's level of pain and possible causes of pain, and understand the medications and methods used to control pain.
- Under the supervision of the kennel manager or a veterinary technician, medicate and treat boarders, including the proper and safe administration of oral, otic, ophthalmic, and topical medications; insulin injections; and subcutaneous fluid therapy. Record treatments on pets' cards and kennel's logs.
- Inform the practice manager or doctors immediately of all bite or scratch wounds you suffer so that reports can be made and you can be referred for timely medical care by a physician, if necessary. Clean all wounds quickly and thoroughly.

Grooming Tasks
- Deflea patients with flea combs, flea sprays, spot-on topicals, baths, dips, or appropriate medication as directed by the kennel manager, veterinary technician, or doctor.
- Detick pets using proper instruments or techniques.
- Trim nails to the quick without causing bleeding.
- Clip and remove matted hair without injuring the underlying skin, and provide other grooming services.
- Administer medicated baths and dips.
- Provide cooling baths for overheated patients under veterinary supervision.

Kennel Procedures and Maintenance Tasks

Patient-Transfer and Record-Keeping Tasks
- Add admitted pets to kennel or hospital logs.
- Coordinate transfers or movement of pets with the front desk and/or veterinarians.
- Maintain accurate kennel records that include the number, type, and locations of boarders, special diets and requirements, your observations of boarders, and treatments or medications administered.
- Advise the front desk when requested services were not provided due to scheduling glitches or inclement weather so that front-desk staff can ensure proper billing.

Cage-Cleaning Tasks

- Follow procedures for cleaning and disinfecting cages and runs.
- Remove feces and place them in a separate container for disposal as directed by the practice or kennel manager.
- Remove food and dirt from cages and runs.
- Clean cages with spray disinfectant and paper towels. Clean runs with disinfectant and a scrub brush or high pressure cleaning system. Wash cages and runs with a dilute (one part bleach to 32 parts water) bleach solution weekly and after occupation by potentially contagious animals.
- Remove and wash all bedding after use. Empty and wash water pails, bowls, and food dishes after use.

Facility-Maintenance Tasks

- Maintain kennel and grounds as directed by the practice or kennel manager. Mow lawns. Tend plantings. Mulch as needed. Periodically treat the grounds to reduce the number of parasites present.
- Ensure safe walkways during inclement weather. Remove ice and/or snow from walkways and runs. Place salt or sand on walkways as needed.
- Gather garbage and place it in designated receptacles.
- Ensure the proper functioning of all kennel equipment. Periodically clean and maintain cleaning, snow-removal, and lawn-care equipment. Repair or replace broken lights and fixtures. Maintain and repair cages and runs to ensure their secure closure and safety. Bring significant malfunctions to the attention of the kennel manager.
- Clean and restock food bins.
- Note low inventory in food, cleaning, and restraint supplies. List items and give the list to the ordering manager.
- Know all the cleaning products used, including their safe handling and proper use.
- Maintain a "lost and found" bin for items left behind by pets' owners. Tag and date each item. Discard or donate items not retrieved after three months.

CHAPTER 9

KENNEL ASSISTANT TRAINING SCHEDULE

Week One

By the end of week one, new kennel assistants should have learned to:

General Knowledge and Tasks

- Follow OSHA standards. Be able to find Material Safety Data Sheets quickly.
- Maintain accurate personal time cards.
- Participate in their performance appraisals, and, as requested, in those of others.
- Participate in all staff and training meetings.

Client-Interaction Tasks

- Administer tick and/or flea repellants or pesticides at the time patients are admitted as directed by the kennel manager.
- Take custody of pets from clients. Restrain dogs with the practice's leashes. Label and store clients' collars and leashes and return them to clients promptly when pets are retrieved from the facility.
- Weigh pets and record weights at the time they are admitted.
- Walk or carry pets to the appropriate wards. Apply facility identification bands. Settle pets comfortably in their assigned cages and runs. Provide fresh water, if permitted, and clean bedding. Identify cages and runs with cage cards. Properly label and place or store personal items left behind by owners.
- Make sure that all kennel and cage doors are properly secured after admitting or moving patients and before leaving the facility at the end of a shift.

- On the day of discharge, gather pets' toys, bedding, and/or food and medications in preparation for discharge.
- Check all pets for cleanliness prior to discharge. Clean, bathe, and/or groom pets prior to discharge as needed. Assess additional fees as directed. Discharge pets and all belongings to clients.
- Measure and record pets' exit weights for comparison against entry weights.

Pet-Care Tasks

- Use warning stickers and notations on cage cards and records as appropriate.
- Follow the practice's procedures and state guidelines in handling suspected or potential rabies cases. Inform the kennel manager, veterinary technicians, or doctors of indications that patients are having difficulty swallowing, exhibiting rear- or front-leg weakness, or showing other neurological changes.
- Wash, dry, and store patients' bedding and the practice's towels. Bedding should be in good repair. Wash surgical towels separately.
- When transferring boarders to new locations, provide them with clean, soft bedding and fresh water.
- Ensure birds and exotic pets' needs and environmental conditions are met, including proper housing, perches, bedding, and diet.
- Walk dogs on a double leash or on a leash within a fenced exercise area. Ensure that they are restrained and under your control at all times.
- Provide individual or group playtime for boarders at clients' request and as directed by the practice or kennel manager. Ensure pets' safety and well-being at all times.
- Prepare meals according to clients', doctors', technicians', or kennel manager's instructions. Feed animals. Note the volume of food eaten or rejected on cage cards or kennel logs.
- Withhold food and water from pets scheduled for or recovering from anesthetic and/or surgical procedures as directed.
- Rinse and refill water pails and dishes at least once daily. Wash and disinfect food and water dishes as needed during pets' stays and after their departure.
- Monitor pets and kennels/cages urine, feces, vomit, and/or blood.

Kennel Procedures and Maintenance Tasks

- Add newly admitted pets to kennel or hospital logs.
- Coordinate transfers or movement of pets with the front desk, technicians, and/or veterinarians.
- Maintain accurate kennel records that include the number, type, and location of boarders, special dietary requirements, your behavioral and medical observations of boarders, and treatments or medications administered.
- Advise the front desk when requested services were not provided due to scheduling glitches or inclement weather so front-desk staff can ensure proper billing.
- Follow procedures for cleaning and disinfecting cages and runs.
- Remove feces and place them in a separate container for disposal as directed by the practice or kennel manager.
- Remove food and dirt from cages and runs.
- Clean cages with spray disinfectant and paper towels. Clean runs with disinfectant and a scrub brush or high-pressure cleaning system. Wash cages and runs with a dilute (one part bleach to 32 parts water) bleach solution weekly and after occupation by potentially contagious animals.
- Remove and wash all bedding after use. Empty and wash water pails, bowls, and food dishes after use.
- Gather garbage and place it in designated receptacles.

Month One

By the end of month one, new kennel assistants should have learned to:

General Knowledge and Tasks

- Know and use standard medical and business and abbreviations.

General Tasks
- Maintain a list of tasks and engage in productive work during slow periods.

- Follow established facility closing procedures to ensure the security of patients, boarders, and the building.

Client-Interaction Tasks

- Cordially greet incoming clients and patients, addressing each by name.
- Check on the immunization status of arriving pets before admitting them to the facility.
- Advise clients of recommended services, such as exercise, play time, larger compartments, and grooming for their pet. Inform them of special call-in times to check on patients or boarders.
- Explain special programs offered by the practice.
- Obtain and record contact information from clients to ensure that they or their agents can be reached during pets' stays.
- Ensure that all boarding admission paperwork has been completed.
- Note special instructions requested by clients.
- Assist clients with unruly or unrestrained pets. Ensure that all dogs are leashed and that cats and smaller pets are caged. Isolate aggressive pets.
- Provide clients with summary evaluations of their pets' boarding stays. Advise them of significant events during their pets' boarding, including changes in anxiety and/or signs of illness, such as constant barking (dogs) or hiding (cats), loss of appetite, diarrhea, excessive thirst, sneezing, or coughing.

Pet-Care Tasks

- Restrain pets in a manner that allows necessary work to be performed, minimizes stress to them, and ensures the safety of pets and people.
- Know and use, when appropriate, various techniques to restrain fractious pets, including:
    1. muzzles, choke collars, Gentle Leader" headcollars, body harnesses, collars, cat bags, and "rabies poles";
    2. blankets, towels, or nets to trap and move cats, dogs, and pocket pets;
    3. collars and lead ropes through cage doors and chain-link fences or over tables; and

4. use of physical restraint using your body, hands, and/or arms.
- Aid veterinarians and technicians in the restraint and evaluation of incoming animals through examinations and health tests. Assist in administering immunizations and parasite treatments.
- Follow isolation procedures for contagious or potentially contagious animals.
- Collect and save urine and fecal samples as requested.
- Know the key symptoms of emergency medical problems likely to be exhibited by boarders. Immediately notify the kennel manager or veterinary staff members if you observe any of the following clinical signs:
    1. Dogs or cats that are unable to or are straining to urinate or defecate
    2. Dogs or cats in heat
    3. Dogs suffering from gastric dilatation and volvulus (GDV or bloat), (i.e., bloated abdomens, unproductive vomiting, vomiting thick ropy saliva, and/or general discomfort)
    4. Difficult, heavy, or rapid breathing
    5. Sneezing, coughing, or ocular discharges
    6. Listlessness
    7. Loss of balance
    8. Inability to rise
    9. Anxiety
    10. Seizures
    11. Significant vomiting and/or diarrhea, especially bloody or foul-smelling diarrhea
    12. Bleeding
- Monitor the behavior of boarders and note potentially aggressive behaviors.
- Identify a patient's level of pain and possible causes of pain, and understand the medications and methods used to control pain.

Kennel Procedures and Maintenance Tasks

- Clean and restock food bins.
- Note low inventory in food, cleaning, and restraint supplies. List the items and give the list to the ordering manager.

- Know all the cleaning products used, including their safe handling and proper use.
- Maintain a "lost and found" bin for items left behind by pets' owners.

Month Three

By the end of month three, new kennel assistants should have learned to:

General Knowledge and Tasks

- Be familiar with infectious diseases, including their prevention and steps to reduce or eliminate transmission. Know the most common zoonotic diseases.
- Answer preliminary questions from interested parties regarding stray and adoptable animals.
- Be prepared to handle any pet or facility emergency that may arise, including dog or cat fights and choking or strangulating animals.

Pet Care Tasks

- Evaluate incoming animals for obvious signs of disease and readily felt skin or body masses or tumors. Find and identify external parasites. Bring noted problems to the attention of pet owners and staff for discussion and resolution prior to admittance.
- Under the supervision of the kennel manager or a veterinary technician, medicate and treat boarders, including the proper and safe administration of oral, otic, ophthalmic, and topical medications; insulin injections; and subcutaneous fluid therapy. Record treatments on pets' cards and kennel's logs.
- Trim nails to the quick without causing bleeding.
- Clip and remove matted hair without injuring the underlying skin.

- Administer medicated baths and dips.
- Provide cooling baths for overheated patients under veterinary supervision.

Kennel Procedures and Maintenance Tasks

- Maintain kennel and grounds as directed by the practice or kennel manager. Mow lawns. Tend plantings. Mulch as needed. Periodically treat the grounds to reduce the number of parasites.
- Ensure safe walkways during inclement weather. Remove ice and snow from walkways and runs. Place salt or sand on walkways as needed.

Month Six

By the end of month six, new kennel assistants should have learned to:

General Knowledge and Tasks

- Be reasonably familiar with breeds and coat colors.
- Use proper medical terminology when speaking and writing.
- Conduct tours of the practice and/or kennel. Before each tour, ensure that the facility is orderly and that staff and patients are prepared for tours.

Client Interaction Tasks

- Advise clients of significant changes in policies or services since their last visit.

Kennel Procedures and Maintenance Tasks

- Ensure the proper functioning of all kennel equipment. Periodically clean and maintain cleaning, snow-removal, and lawn-care equipment. Repair or replace broken lights and fixtures. Maintain and repair cages and runs to ensure their secure closure and safety.

CHAPTER 10

KENNEL MANAGER JOB DESCRIPTION

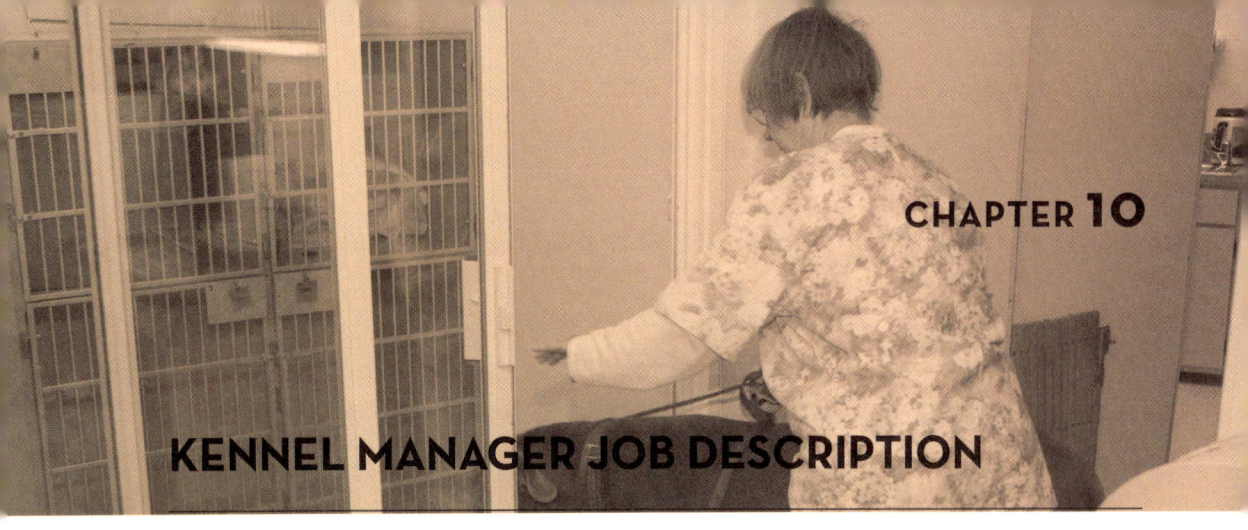

Veterinary practice kennel managers have the primary responsibility for greeting clients; admitting pets to the boarding facility; and feeding, handling, and cleaning up after boarding animals. In many practices, they will have secondary responsibilities to assist with the care of hospitalized animals. Kennel managers must select, hire, train, supervise, evaluate, and discipline kennel staff members.

In addition, kennel managers establish protocols, handle food and supplies inventories, organize and assist with facility maintenance, and, in some practices, provide direct nursing care for pets. The position requires a high school diploma, patience and experience working with animals and people, confidence working with difficult and sometimes aggressive pets, sufficient business aptitude and skills to handle the financial affairs of the kennel, and an aptitude for and the skills to maintain and repair the kennel facility.

General Knowledge and Tasks

General Knowledge

- Be reasonably familiar with dog and cat breeds and coat colors.
- Follow OSHA standards. Be able to find Material Safety Data Sheets quickly.
- Know and use basic medical abbreviations.
- Use proper medical terminology when speaking and writing.
- Be familiar with infectious diseases, including their prevention and steps to reduce or eliminate transmission. Know the most common zoonotic diseases.
- Competently speak and write the English language.
- Competently speak a second language commonly used at the practice.

General Tasks

- Develop and post a personal work schedule so that others will know when you are available. In addition to scheduled hours, provide home and mobile contact phone numbers and be available as additional duties and emergency circumstances demand.
- Arrive for work punctually so as to set a good example for kennel staff.
- Maintain accurate personal time cards.
- Maintain a professional appearance while at work, including clean and pressed uniforms or clothes. Change clothes daily as necessary to look professional and avoid carrying odors.
- Smile and maintain an even, friendly demeanor while on the job. Perform job tasks efficiently without rushing.
- Handle stress and pressure with poise and tact.
- Show respect for clients, team members, and animals (alive or deceased) at all times.
- Have the physical strength and ability to stand for an entire shift when needed, and be able to lift pets and objects weighing up to 50 pounds without assistance, handle repetitive up-and-down or back-and-forth motions, and work while bending. Assist in lifting patients weighing more than 50 pounds.
- Keep up with new developments in the field through journals and continuing education. Attend off-site continuing education as requested by the manager or owner(s).
- Participate in your performance appraisal and, as requested, in those of others.
- Handle communications with staff, doctors, clients, detail reps, and vendors with a professional demeanor.
- Conduct tours of the practice and/or kennel. Before each tour, ensure that the facility is orderly and that staff and patients are prepared for tours.
- Maintain constant vigilance regarding open doorways that could allow pets to escape from the facility.
- Maintain strict confidentiality regarding clients and patients for whom the practice provides veterinary services.
- Be prepared to handle any pet or facility emergency that may arise, including dog or cat fights, choking or strangulating animals, and facility fire or weather-related emergencies. Follow contingency plans.
- Follow established facility closing procedures to ensure the security of patients, boarders, and the building.

CLIENT-INTERACTION TASKS

PATIENT-ADMITTANCE TASKS

- Cordially greet incoming clients and pets, addressing each by name.
- Check on the immunization status of all arriving pets. Make recommendations to clients regarding vaccine status, and enforce preventative-care requirements in accordance with the practice's and kennel's policies and standards.
- Advise clients of specific call-in times to check on hospitalized patients or boarders as well as recommended services, such as the availability and cost for larger quarters for boarders, options for exercise and play time, opportunities for obedience training and grooming, and/or the provision of medical services while boarding.
- Explain special programs offered by the practice.
- Advise clients of significant changes in policies or services since their last visit.
- Answer preliminary questions from interested parties regarding stray and adoptable animals. Develop and handle the paperwork for adoptions. (For well-conceived adoption-consent forms, see pages 66–67 of AAHA Press's *Legal Consent Forms for Veterinary Practices*.)
- Obtain and record contact information from clients to ensure that they or their agents can be reached during their pets' stays.
- Ensure that all boarding admission paperwork has been completed. (For examples of boarding agreements, see pages 64–66 of AAHA Press's *Legal Consent Forms for Veterinary Practices*.)
- Assist clients with unruly or unrestrained pets. Ensure that all dogs are leashed and that cats and smaller pets are caged. Develop and implement a plan to isolate aggressive pets in a manner and in a location that prevents harm to other boarders or staff members. Request assistance if needed.
- Take custody of pets from clients. Restrain dogs with the practice's leashes. Label and store clients' collars and leashes and return them to clients promptly when pets are retrieved from the facility.
- Note special care instructions given by clients, and ensure that such requests are fulfilled.
- Weigh pets and record weights at the time they are admitted.

- Walk or carry pets to the appropriate wards or kennels. Apply identification bands. Settle pets comfortably in their assigned cages and runs. Provide fresh water, if permitted, and clean bedding. Mark cages and runs with pets' cage cards. Properly label and place or store personal items left behind by owners.
- Use warning stickers and notations on cage cards and records as appropriate.
- Aid veterinarians and technicians with the evaluation of incoming animals through physical examinations and health tests. Assist in administering immunizations and parasite treatments.
- Recognize the symptoms of contagious diseases. Follow isolation procedures for contagious or potentially contagious animals. Using designated products and dilutions for disinfectants, properly disinfect your shoes, hands, and clothing before leaving isolation areas.
- Follow the practice's procedures and state guidelines when handling suspected or potential rabies cases. Inform doctors of signs that patients are having difficulty swallowing, exhibiting leg weakness, or exhibiting other neurologic signs.
- Ensure that all kennel and cage doors are properly secured after admitting or moving pets and before leaving the facility at the end of a shift.

PATIENT-DISCHARGE TASKS
- Develop and use materials to provide clients with summary evaluations of their pets' boarding stays. Advise them of significant events during their pets' boarding, including changes in anxiety and/or signs of illness, such as constant barking (dogs) or hiding (cats), loss of appetite, weight loss, diarrhea, excessive thirst, sneezing, or coughing.
- On the day of discharge, gather pets' toys, bedding, medications, and food in preparation for discharge.
- Check all pets for cleanliness prior to discharge. Clean, bathe, and/or groom pets prior to discharge as needed. Assess additional fees as directed. Discharge pets.
- Measure and record pets' exit weights for comparison against their entry weights.
- Assist doctors in locating and, at the direction of a doctor, calling clients to inform them of the deaths of their pets while

boarding. Use extraordinary care and compassion when communicating with a client if the pet's death was unexpected.
- Handle angry or grieving clients in a calm and reassuring manner. Keep information about grief counselors and provide it to clients in need.
- Assist clients to their cars if needed.

Pet-Care Tasks

Examination and Restraint Tasks

- Restrain pets in a manner that allows necessary work to be performed, minimizes stress to pets, and ensures the safety of pets and people.
- Evaluate incoming animals for obvious signs of disease, readily felt skin or body tumors, and the presence of external parasites. Bring noted problems to the attention of pet owners and staff for discussion and resolution prior to admittance.
- Know and use, when appropriate, various techniques to restrain fractious pets, including:
    1. muzzles, choke collars, Gentle Leader" headcollars, body harnesses, collars, cat bags, and "rabies poles";
    2. blankets, towels, or nets to trap and move cats, dogs, and pocket pets;
    3. collars and lead ropes through cage doors and chain-link fences or over tables; and
    4. use of physical restraint using your body, hands, and/or arms.

Pet-Care and Grooming Tasks

- Work with the front desk and practice manager to care for and return stray or abandoned animals to their owners, or legally find them new homes.
- Wash, dry, and store patients' bedding and the practice's towels. Bedding should be in good repair. Wash surgical towels separately.
- Maximize pets' comfort with a gentle and reassuring manner. Understand that actions that would constitute animal cruelty under state or local laws or the practice's policies will be grounds for immediate reprimand and/or termination.

- Monitor boarders for illness outbreaks and trends. Whenever possible, determine cause of illness. With input from veterinary staff, change procedures to minimize ongoing or future disease.
- Identify a patient's level of pain and possible causes of pain, and understand the medications and methods used to control pain.
- When transferring boarders to new locations, provide them with clean, soft bedding and fresh water.
- Walk dogs on a double leash or on a leash within a fenced exercise area. Ensure that they are restrained and under your control at all times.
- Provide individual or group play time for boarders at clients' request. Ensure pets' safety and well-being at all times.
- Prepare meals according to clients' or doctors' instructions, and feed animals. Note the volume of food eaten or rejected on cage cards or kennel logs.
- Withhold food and water for appropriate time periods from pets scheduled for or recovering from surgical procedures and anesthesia as directed.
- Rinse and refill water pails and dishes at least once daily. Wash and disinfect as needed during and after the completion of pets' stays.
- Monitor pets and kennels/cages urine, feces, vomit, and blood. When noted, clean pets and cages or runs immediately. Note incidents on cage cards or kennel logs. Bring signs of illnesses to the attention of staff doctors as indicated.
- Collect and save urine and fecal samples as requested.
- Continuously monitor pets under your care. Pay particular attention to signs of distress, illness, or injury.
- Know the key symptoms of emergency medical problems likely to be exhibited by boarders. Immediately notify veterinary staff members if you observe any of the following clinical signs:
    1. Dogs or cats that are unable to or are straining to urinate or defecate
    2. Dogs or cats in heat
    3. Dogs suffering from gastric dilatation and volvulus (GDV or bloat), (i.e., bloated abdomens, unproductive vomiting, vomiting thick ropy saliva, and/or general discomfort)
    4. Difficult, heavy, or rapid breathing
    5. Sneezing, coughing, or ocular discharges
    6. Listlessness

7. Loss of balance
8. Inability to rise
9. Anxiety
10. Seizures
11. Significant vomiting and/or diarrhea, especially bloody or foul-smelling diarrhea
12. Bleeding

- Monitor boarders' behaviors and note potential aggressive behaviors. Use caution when handling aggressive or potentially aggressive pets. Request assistance when needed.
- Per kennel policy, administer tick and/or flea repellants or pesticides at the time boarders are admitted.
- Deflea patients with flea combs, flea sprays, spot-on topicals, baths, dips, or appropriate medication based on the health of the patient and in accordance with the kennel's policies.
- Detick patients.
- Trim nails to the quick without causing bleeding.
- Provide medical grooming, including medicated baths, dips, nail trims, and mat removal.
- Provide cooling baths for heatstroke patients under veterinary supervision.
- Medicate and treat boarders. Properly and safely administer oral, otic, ophthalmic, and topical medications. Accurately administer insulin injections and subcutaneous fluid therapy. Record treatments on pets' cards, kennel's logs, or medical records. Request assistance from veterinary technicians when handling difficult pets or unfamiliar treatments.
- Inform the practice manager or doctors immediately of all bite or scratch wounds you suffer so that reports can be made and you can be referred for timely medical care by a physician, if necessary. Clean all wounds quickly and thoroughly.
- Maintain bodies of deceased pets in accordance with kennel policies.

Kennel Procedures and Maintenance Tasks

- Add newly admitted pets to kennel or hospital logs.
- Coordinate transfers or movement of pets with the front desk and/or veterinarians.

- Maintain accurate kennel records that include the number, type, and location of boarders, special diets and requirements, observations of boarders, and treatments or medications administered.
- Advise the front desk when requested services were not provided due to scheduling glitches or inclement weather so that front-desk staff can ensure proper billing.

Cage-Cleaning Tasks

- Follow procedures for cleaning and disinfecting cages and runs.
- Remove feces and place them in a separate container for disposal as directed by the practice or kennel manager.
- Remove food and dirt from cages and runs.
- Clean cages with spray disinfectant and paper towels. Clean runs with disinfectant and a scrub brush or high- pressure cleaning system. Wash cages and runs with a dilute (one part bleach to 32 parts water) bleach solution weekly and after occupation by potentially contagious animals.
- Remove and wash all bedding after use. Empty and wash water pails, bowls, and food dishes after use.

Facility-Maintenance Tasks

- Maintain kennel and grounds. Mow lawns. Tend plantings. Mulch as needed. Periodically treat the grounds to reduce the number of parasites present.
- Ensure safe walkways during inclement weather. Remove ice and snow from walkways and runs. Place salt or sand on walkways as required.
- Gather garbage and place it in designated receptacles.
- Ensure the proper functioning of all equipment. Periodically clean and maintain cleaning, snow-removal, and lawn-care equipment. Repair or replace broken lights and fixtures. Maintain and repair cages and runs to ensure their secure closure and safety.
- Clean food bins as needed, but at least monthly. Restock food bins.
- Know all the cleaning products used, including their safe handling and proper use.
- Maintain a "lost and found" bin for items left behind by pets' owners. Tag and date each item. Discard or donate items not retrieved after three months.

Managerial Tasks

General Managerial Tasks

- Develop and use kennel forms, including kennel logs, daily and weekly checklists, cage cards, admittance forms, and boarding "report cards."
- Develop, or assist in the development of, and continually evaluate protocols for:
  1. Admitting boarders
  2. Cleaning procedures
  3. Isolating infectious animals
  4. Disease outbreaks
  5. Exercising boarders
  6. Food storage and distribution
  7. Discharging guests
  8. Closing and security procedures
- Develop written procedures for, train others in, and follow protocols for handling:
  1. Animal emergencies
  2. Pets that have escaped from the facility
  3. Employees who have been bitten or scratched
  4. Natural disasters, including fires, floods, hurricanes, and tornados
  5. Internal emergencies, including power losses, fires, and dangerous persons
  6. Man-made disasters necessitating rapid exit from the property
- Schedule kennel staff to ensure adequate coverage while minimizing downtime, overstaffing, and overtime.
- Promote a positive attitude among staff.
- Manage inventory so that items are consistently in stock. Ensure that the least possible amounts of money and space are dedicated to kennel inventory. Establish standard inventory stocks of food, cleaning agents, water containers, bedding, litter and litter pans, leashes, pet carriers, and paper towels.
- Work with the practice manager to establish an annual kennel budget. Follow the budget when making purchasing and staffing decisions. Discuss budget adjustments with the practice manager, and make recommendations regarding boarding fees that will ensure the profitability of the kennel.

- Investigate complaints. Resolve complaints in a manner that supports the practice's mission and policies. When appropriate, advise complainants of your resolutions.
- Mediate disputes between kennel staff and others. Ensure that all sides are fairly heard and considered and that the dispute resolution is just.
- Develop friendly, professional relationships with boarding clients.
- Develop and implement value-added services for boarders. Develop special programs and marketing materials to enhance clients' experiences, boarders' experiences, client retention, and the kennel's visibility within the community.

Hiring Tasks

- Recruit new employees by posting notices, placing classified advertisements, attending job fairs, and via direct solicitation. Create advertisements for staff positions and determine where to advertise to most effectively fill vacancies.
- Review job applications and resumes for kennel personnel. Conduct phone and/or in-person interviews of potential employees. Assess their personalities, intelligence, potential for loyalty and care-giving, enthusiasm, stability, judgment, and technical skills. Check references and, if appropriate, run credit, drug, and background checks.
- When applicants will not be offered employment, inform them within a reasonable time period.
- Offer successful applicants employment and provide details of the offer, including start date, initial salary, and benefits. Once the offer has been accepted, ensure that paperwork for newly hired staff members has been completed, including:
    1. Payroll information
    2. I-9 verification of work eligibility
    3. W-9 tax withholding
    4. Health-coverage applications
    5. Other fringe benefits forms
- Provide new hires with job descriptions and performance-appraisal forms. Clearly define expectations.

Training Tasks

- Train new and existing kennel staff to:

1. Follow OSHA guidelines
2. Protect boarders, patients, and staff from infectious diseases and other health risks
3. Reduce or eliminate the hazards of physical kennel work
4. Follow kennel procedures
5. Secure boarders and the kennel facility
6. Clean facility
7. Maintain grounds
8. Feed and give water to pets
9. Recognize signs of distress and disease
10. Properly medicate and treat pets
11. Recognize aggression and other problem behaviors
12. Properly restrain pets

- Ensure that procedures and policies are followed.
- Attend and participate in all staff and training meetings.
- Be willing and able to teach other staff members kennel skills. Keep records of all training meetings.
- Supervise kennel employees. Establish work priorities for staff members under your supervision. Ensure that work is completed in a proper, professional, and timely manner. Maintain an efficient workflow. Seek out opportunities to further train or retrain employees.

Performance-Appraisal and Termination Tasks

- Regularly evaluate the job performance of kennel staff and, if requested, the job performance of other staff members. Follow guidelines and use appraisal forms to review and evaluate employees' performances. Teach employees to productively and actively participate in their reviews.
- With the assistance of the practice manager and/or practice owner(s), initiate disciplinary actions against kennel employees. Provide verbal or written warnings for inappropriate work-related behavior, and clearly state the consequences for continued problems. With the agreement of the practice manager, place employees on probation or suspension for serious or chronic work-related offenses. Document actions, and advise the practice manager and/or owner(s).
- Terminate the employment of kennel employees when justified. Conduct exit interviews. Retrieve keys and all property that

belongs to the practice. Advise employees of COBRA options, severance pay, and ongoing benefits as appropriate. Document the circumstances of terminations and exit conversations, and advise the practice manager and/or owner(s).

CHAPTER 11

OFFICE MANAGER JOB DESCRIPTION

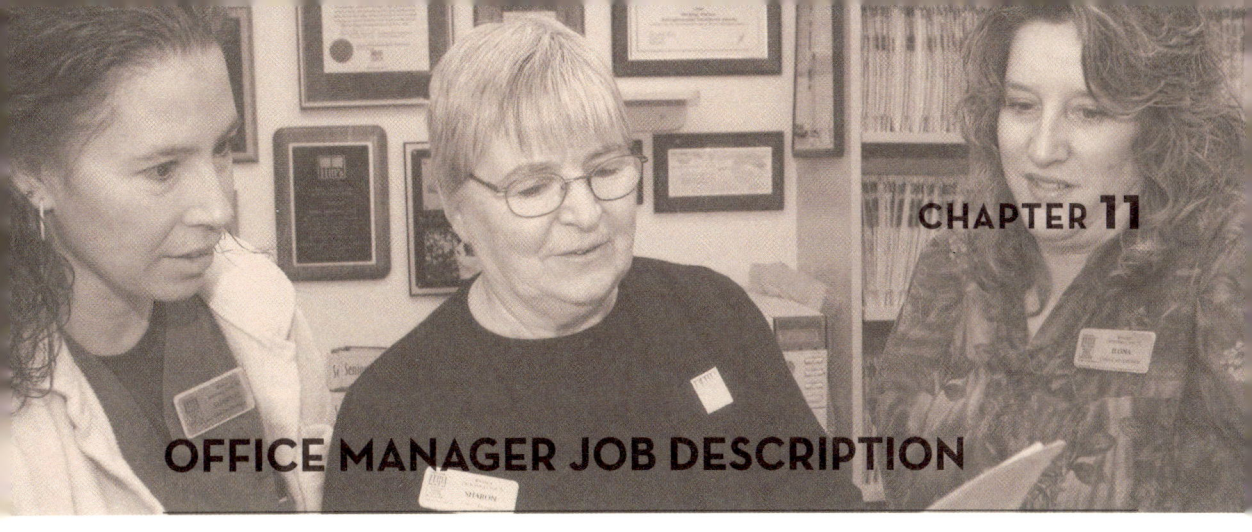

Under the direction and supervision of the practice owner(s) and/or the practice manager, a veterinary practice's office manager is responsible for organizing, training, and supervising the front-office staff, including veterinary receptionists, assistants, and bookkeepers. Tasks include establishing protocols for scheduling appointments; creating and maintaining medical records; managing the practice's client and patient database; receiving, handling, and depositing the practice's revenue; and handling the business's accounts receivable.

Office managers must provide effective leadership, assist and support the practice manager, and handle customer and community relations. Office managers should possess a college degree or a minimum of twelve semester hours of business-related course material, and have a minimum of two years' office-management experience.

General Knowledge and Tasks

General Knowledge
- Be reasonably familiar with breeds and coat colors.
- Follow OSHA standards. Be able to find Material Safety Data Sheets quickly.
- Know and use basic medical abbreviations.
- Use proper medical terminology when speaking and writing.
- Competently speak and write the English language.
- Competently speak a second language commonly used at the practice.

General Tasks
- Develop and post a personal work schedule so that others will know when you are available. In addition to scheduled hours, provide home and mobile contact phone numbers, and be available as additional duties and emergency circumstances demand.

- Arrive for work punctually so as to set a good example for staff.
- Maintain accurate personal time cards.
- Maintain a professional appearance while at work, including clean and pressed uniforms or clothes. Change clothes daily as necessary to look professional and avoid carrying odors.
- Smile and maintain an even, friendly demeanor while on the job. Perform job tasks efficiently without rushing.
- Handle stress and pressure with poise and tact.
- Show respect for clients, team members, and animals (alive or deceased) at all times.
- Have the physical strength and ability to lift pets and objects weighing up to 50 pounds without assistance. Assist in lifting patients weighing more than 50 pounds.
- Participate in your performance appraisal.
- Handle communications with staff, doctors, clients, detail reps, and vendors with a professional demeanor.
- Conduct tours of the practice and/or kennel. Before each tour, ensure that the facility is orderly and that staff and patients are prepared for tours.
- Maintain constant vigilance regarding open doorways that could allow pets to escape from the facility.
- Maintain strict confidentiality regarding clients and patients for whom the practice provides veterinary services.
- Be prepared to handle any pet or facility emergency that may arise, including dog or cat fights, choking or strangulating animals, and facility fire or weather-related emergencies. Follow contingency plans.
- Follow established closing procedures to ensure the security of patients, staff, data, revenue, inventory, and the facility.

Client-Interaction Tasks

- Use clients' and patients' names during conversations.
- Provide basic pricing information to client phone inquiries. Respond in a manner that encourages potential clients to visit the practice.
- Offer financial estimates to clients for services as directed by doctors. Teach other support staff how to handle this task with confidence and tact.

- Counsel clients on payment options. Enlist doctors or veterinary technicians to answer medical questions or questions requiring medical judgment beyond your expertise.
- Discuss and enforce policies regarding payments, credit, pet health insurance, and finance fees. Assist with CareCredit® applications.
- File pet insurance claims on behalf of clients.
- Review various legal-consent forms with clients, explain them, answer questions, and have clients sign the forms. Check that clients' signatures match the signatures on the records.
- Advise clients of recommended services for their pets.
- Explain special programs offered by the practice.
- Place special diet or product orders at clients' requests. Advise clients of prices, including shipping and handling fees and expected delivery dates. Ensure that clients are called when special orders arrive.
- Advise clients of significant changes in policies or services since their last visit.
- Provide clients with handouts and brochures explaining relevant medical conditions, surgeries, immunizations, internal and external parasites, pet insurance, and diets.
- Explain delays that may affect clients. Keep clients and patients comfortable during the time they are waiting for service.
- Placate and/or compensate clients distressed by long waits, scheduling glitches, and other problems.
- Handle angry or grieving clients with a calm and reassuring manner. Be familiar with the grieving process. Always be sensitive to background chatter or conversations that could exacerbate the anxieties and grief clients experience during euthanasias or deaths of their pets.
- Provide or arrange for grief counseling for clients in need.
- Inform the practice manager or doctors immediately of all bite or scratch wounds you suffer so that reports can be made and you can be referred for timely medical care by a physician, if necessary. Clean all wounds quickly and thoroughly.

Office-Management Tasks

General Office-Management Tasks

- Arrange for the production and distribution of business cards for veterinarians and staff members.
- Understand how to operate all office business machines, including fax machines, copiers, personal digital assistants (PDAs), pagers, and voice-mail or messaging systems.
- Plan, develop, and coordinate policies and procedures for:
  1. Keeping medical records;
  2. Ordering, receiving, and inventorying drugs and supplies
  3. Scheduling shifts for staff
  4. Front-office opening and closing procedures
  5. Recording and storing employee time sheets
  6. Creating and implementing effective client-reminder systems
- Ensure that service reminders and thank-you, welcome, condolence, and birthday cards are all sent in a timely manner.
- Deliver deposits to the bank daily or as directed, ensuring that the person who completed the deposit slip is different than the person making the bank deposit.
- Develop, train others in, and follow protocols for handling:
  1. Animal emergencies
  2. Pets that have escaped from the facility
  3. Employees who have been bitten or scratched
  4. Natural disasters, including fires, flooding, hurricanes, and tornados
  5. Internal emergencies, including power losses, fires, and dangerous persons
  6. Man-made disasters necessitating rapid exit from the property
- Investigate complaints. As stipulated by the owner(s) or practice manager, seek input from these parties as needed. Resolve complaints in a manner that best supports the practice's mission and philosophy. When appropriate, advise complainants of your findings and the resolutions of the complaints.
- Mediate disputes between receptionists and others. Ensure that all sides are fairly heard, that facts are properly gathered and documented, that the dispute resolution is fair and just, and that legal counsel is sought as needed.
- Evaluate general-business, health, professional liability, worker's compensation, and/or company-auto insurance policies yearly.

Ensure that coverage is current and complete. Periodically seek quotes from alternate companies for comparison.
- Be familiar with federal and state regulations regarding pharmacy, controlled-drug, and staffing issues.
- Gather and compile data to assist the practice manager in preparing financial and business reports.

Front-Desk Tasks
- Open, date stamp, sort, and distribute mail.
- Know and perform receptionist duties when necessary.
- Ensure that the doctors, technicians, and assistants enter occupied exam rooms within reasonable time periods.
- Arrange for waiting-room amenities, such as current magazines, beverages, telephone, and/or television.
- Maintain a file of lost and found pets.
- Maintain contact information for and communications with animal-control officers, animal inspectors, or town officials regarding lost or stray animals and animals subject to rabies quarantines.
- Develop and/or maintain a list of local resources for obedience training, behavior, boarding, and grooming services.

Phone Tasks
- Know phone functions, including hold, intercom, transfer, forward, and three-way calling.
- Arrange for a reliable and cordial answering service, and provide the service's staff with specific, complete instructions for appropriate greetings, triage, and doctor-on-call contacts.
- Establish an appropriate message on the answering machine.
- Ensure that calls are transferred to the answering machine or answering service during staff meetings and closed hours.

Computer and Internet Tasks
- Program the practice-management software to maintain and search for, store, and print specialized lists from the database, such as:
    1. Patients that are overdue for services
    2. Clients with past due or overdue balances on their accounts

3. New patient/client lists
4. Numbers of new clients per month
5. Average client-transaction or invoice fees (ACTs)
6. Income production by doctor and by groomer
7. Doctors' average client-transaction or invoice fees (Dr. ACTs)

- Draft letters and modify and print forms or letters for clients.
- Generate records of rabies immunizations for clients and for town, city, and county officials.
- Assign computer passwords and identification codes to veterinarians and staff members. Ensure they are properly used so that employees' work can be audited and entries are properly attributed to veterinarians and staff members.
- Access and navigate the Internet to find veterinary websites, order supplies, and access information for clients.
- Assist with or supervise website design and changes.
- Assign and maintain email accounts. Check email regularly for clients' questions, requests, and information. Reply to emails or pass them on to appropriate employees.
- Back up computer files at the close of each business day, and ensure the backup is transported and secured at a location off the premises.

Forms, Handouts, and Medical-Record Tasks

- Work with practice manager, doctors, and/or practice owners to develop templates for descriptions of procedures and associated fees. See Resources section at the end of this manual for a source for this information.
- Develop and use:
  1. Admittance forms
  2. Disclaimers and legal consent forms
  3. New client and patient forms
  4. Inventory-control forms
  5. Time records
- Draft, seek editorial review for, and publish brochures and handouts. Periodically evaluate the publications for accuracy and contemporary nature of the data; update as necessary.
- Develop and maintain an efficient medical record management system. Ensure that files are filed accurately and found quickly.

Maintain specific locations or storage bins where active and inactive files are stored.

Human-Resource Management Tasks

General Human-Resource Tasks

- Promote a positive attitude among staff.
- Schedule staff to ensure adequate coverage while minimizing downtime and overtime.
- Develop personnel policies and a personnel policy manual that set standards for:
    1. Hiring
    2. Staff training
    3. Performance appraisals
    4. Fringe benefits
    5. Pay
    6. Work schedules
    7. Vacations
    8. Jury duty
    9. Maternity and other leaves of absence
    10. Holiday schedules and pay
    11. Overtime
    12. Continuing education
    13. Sick pay
    14. Disabilities
    15. Complaints regarding discrimination
    16. Complaints regarding sexual harassment
    17. Legal notifications
    18. Tardiness
    19. Personal time
    20. Disciplinary action
    21. Employment terminations
- Reevaluate and revise policies and the employee manual as needed. (Note: AAHA offers the *AAHA Guide to Creating an Employee Handbook*, Second Edition to help you accomplish this task.)

- Establish and maintain accurate employee records files in a locked filing cabinet. Protect the confidentiality of such information.

Hiring Tasks

- Develop and use job applications for various staff positions.
- Recruit new employees by posting notices, placing classified advertisements, attending job fairs, and via direct solicitation. Create advertisements for staff positions and determine where to advertise to most effectively fill vacancies.
- Review job applications and resumes. Conduct phone and/or in-person interviews of potential employees. Assess their personalities, intelligence, potential for loyalty and care-giving, enthusiasm, stability, judgment, and technical skills. Check references and, if appropriate, run credit, drug, and background checks.
- When applicants will not be offered employment, inform them within a reasonable time period.
- Offer successful applicants employment and provide details of the offer, including start date, initial salary, and benefits. Once the offer has been accepted, complete the new-hire paperwork, including:
    1. Payroll information
    2. I-9 verification of work eligibility
    3. W-9 tax withholding;
    4. Health-coverage applications
    5. Other fringe benefits forms
- Provide new hires with job descriptions and performance-appraisal forms. Clearly define expectations.

Training Tasks

- Train new and existing receptionist staff to follow front-office procedures and OSHA guidelines. Keep records of all training meetings. (Note: AAHA Press offers the *Veterinary Receptionist's Training Manual* available in hard copy and in word-processing software on CD.)
- Supervise receptionists and veterinary assistants, and, as directed by the practice manager, other employees. Establish work priorities for staff members under your supervision. Ensure that work is completed in a proper, professional, and timely manner.

Maintain an efficient workflow. Seek out opportunities to further train or retrain employees.
- Locate commercially available or develop in-house staff-training materials that expedite the training of staff in effective and cost-efficient manners.
- Participate in and/or organize staff and training meetings. Be willing and able to teach computer skills, inventory-management skills, and client-relation skills to other staff members.

Performance-Appraisal and Termination Tasks
- Regularly evaluate the job performance of reception staff and, if requested, the job performance of other staff members. Follow guidelines and use appraisal forms to review and evaluate employees' performances. Teach employees to productively and actively participate in their reviews. (Note: AAHA Press offers *A Practical Guide to Performance Appraisals*.)
- With the assistance of the practice manager and/or the practice's owner(s), initiate disciplinary actions against employees. Provide verbal or written warnings for inappropriate work-related behaviors, and clearly state consequences for continued problems. With the agreement of the practice manager and/or owner(s), place employees on probation or suspension for serious or chronic work offenses. Document actions, and advise the practice manager and/or owner(s).
- Terminate the employment of employees when justified. Conduct exit interviews. Retrieve keys and all property that belongs to the practice. Advise employees of COBRA options, severance pay, and ongoing benefits as appropriate. Document the circumstances of terminations and exit conversations, and advise the practice manager and/or owner(s).

Pay and Benefit Tasks
- Set pay levels for front-office staff and, if requested, for other positions. Establish clear, differentiating skill sets for different pay levels.
- Develop, implement, and manage incentive programs that will bond employees to the practice, encourage superior work performance, and keep costs within the budget allocated for staff expenses. Collect and evaluate data for incentive bonus programs. Distribute bonuses in a timely fashion.

- Determine each doctor's income production, calculate production-based pay, and ensure the distribution of reconciled compensation for doctors at the appropriate time intervals.
- Oversee payroll. Process time records. Adjust records and pay to account for time taken off due to continuing education, vacation, illness, maternity/paternity leave, personal time, and/or disability. Ensure timely delivery or automatic deposits of employee paychecks.
- Administer employee benefits and complete paperwork. Ensure that employees are aware of the benefits available to them. Enroll new employees in benefits programs. Serve as liaison between employees and benefits companies as needed. Deduct established copayments from employees' pay.

Facility and Equipment Tasks

- Ensure regulatory compliance with OSHA, DEA, the State Labor Code, and the state's board of veterinary medicine. Post required agency forms, records, and reports.
- Maintain a file of equipment, instruments, furnishings, and product purchase receipts, instruction booklets, and warranties to ensure easy access.
- Maintain a list of contractors, vendors, and service people for repairs, maintenance work, and emergencies.
- Price, evaluate, and purchase product service or maintenance agreements in accordance with practice manager or owner(s).
- Maintain front-office equipment, including telephones, computers, printers, copiers, calculators, fax machines, music and marketing for telephones "on hold," intercom, electronic credit-card deposit machines, postage meters, security systems, pagers, pencil sharpeners, and digital or video cameras.
- Understand the practice-management software. Serve as a resource to staff for training and for resolving computer problems. Contact customer support if needed.
- Study, price, and inform the practice manager or owner(s) of updates for computer hardware and software to maximize the efficiency of the computer system. Install and maintain upgrades. Train staff on upgrades, or arrange for training to ensure a smooth transition.

- Routinely inspect the facility, grounds, and landscaping to ensure continuous upkeep and maintenance of the buildings and grounds.
- Ensure that the security system is operating properly.

Financial-Management Tasks

- Protect the business from economic losses due to theft, embezzlement, and negligence by developing internal controls to monitor client and bank deposits, payments, and accounts receivable. Maintain tight inventory controls. Carry insurance to protect against theft and embezzlement.
- Prepare monthly and yearly financial and business reports. Present reports to the practice manager or owner(s).
- With the practice manager and/or owner, establish policies regarding client credit, payment schedules, held checks, and finance fees.
- With the practice manager and/or owner(s), evaluate and adjust fees at no less than six-month intervals.
- Maintain accurate business records for all revenues, expenses, and loans.
- Establish and/or maintain a credit application and management system for client accounts.
- Record NSF returned checks in the bookkeeping system and in clients' business records. Adjust clients' accounts by the amounts of checks and returned-check fees. Notify clients of deficiencies by phone or mail.
- Develop and manage a system to track and ensure timely payments on accounts receivable.
- Send monthly invoices updated with finance charges. Properly record payments received.
- Make timely phone reminders on accounts past due, or assign lists of such accounts to doctors who handled the cases, so they can contact the parties before accounts are turned over to a collection agency.
- Follow established legal requirements when communicating with clients.
- Research and, with the aid of the practice manager or owner(s), select a collection agency or attorney to handle severely delinquent accounts. Transfer accounts with no activity that are

greater than ninety days past due to the collection agency, or as directed.
- Track accounts payable and prepare checks, or ensure that the bookkeeper prepares checks, in a timely fashion for the practice manager's or owner's signature. Take advantage of time-sensitive discounts and avoid late fees, disruption in service, or deterioration of relationships with vendors. Handle reimbursements to staff for travel, continuing education, and other approved miscellaneous expenses.
- Maintain a preset amount of petty cash to use for minor daily cash needs. Track petty-cash expenditures and reconcile this account no less than once monthly.
- Ensure that credit-card receipts match statements of credit-card income and that credit-card debits are only for legitimate client refunds. Confirm that cash and check totals match receipts recorded as paid by cash and check, respectively. Investigate and resolve discrepancies, or bring them to the practice owner's or manager's attention immediately.
- Ensure cash drawers are balanced daily.
- Ensure sufficient change and reduce the cash drawer to a preset daily amount at the conclusion of each shift, or train and arrange for another staff person to do this in your absence. Change money at the bank as necessary.
- Oversee the deposit of each day's cash and check income in the proper bank account(s) in a manner that prevents the same staff member from filling out the deposit slips and making the bank deposits.
- Check credit-company statements to ensure that all credits and debits are accurately recorded in the practice's account.
- Correspond with and learn from the CPA. Provide the CPA with essential financial records. Respond to inquiries, and provide additional information when requested.
- Review and reconcile financial reports, ledgers, and budgets.
- Assist the practice manager and the CPA with fiscal planning, including cash-flow needs, debt repayment, and capital investments.
- Provide historical information to the practice manager and assist in developing budgets. Recommend budgets for the front office and inventory that minimize costs while maximizing the value of those expenditures.

- Follow budgets when making purchasing and staffing decisions. Discuss budget adjustments with the practice manager.
- Track payable taxes. With the assistance of the CPA, complete and file accurate monthly, quarterly, and annual tax reports.
- Audit the work of the front-office staff and their adherence to procedures. Ensure that procedures are properly followed and that they are effective.

Inventory-Management Tasks

- Oversee and maintain the drug, vaccine, and hospital and janitorial supply inventory.
- Establish an effective inventory-turnover tracking system so that the practice devotes minimal money and space to store inventory items.
- Develop and/or implement an inventory-control system that minimizes theft by employees or clients.
- Develop minimum drug and hospital supply values and reorder points with the practice manager and doctors. Train staff to properly use the inventory system, and monitor it for correct use.
- Establish and/or maintain a computerized tracking system for accurately inventorying products and supplies.
- Develop purchase orders using computerized inventory data, hand counts, and/or staff's lists of "short" items. Write, track, and file purchase orders.
- Place orders for supplies in a timely fashion. Compare prices and programs from different vendors to ensure the best value on purchases.
- Maintain positive relationships with vendors.
- Discuss new products with detail reps or suppliers. Relay information to veterinarians and the practice manager, and arrange for further communication with company reps or decide which new products to order.
- Know when to take advantage of cost-effective, special-purchase promotions.
- Supervise the receipt of supplies that have been ordered.
- Instruct and oversee staff members as to how they should:

1. Check orders against purchase orders and packing slips to ensure that shipments are accurate upon arrival.
2. Check for breakage or other problems that would render merchandise unusable.
3. Report problems to suppliers.
4. Enter merchandise items into the practice's computerized inventory system.
- Stock office supplies so that materials are consistently available.

Marketing Tasks

- Build friendly, professional relationships with clients, detail reps, and vendors.
- Develop programs and marketing materials that retain clients, enhance their experiences, and increase visibility within the community.
- Develop, plan, and implement special projects, including open houses, pet fairs, pet-week promotions, and school tours and visits.
- Establish and maintain signs that promote visibility, enhance the practice's appearance, and notify clients of important policies.
- Develop, seek contributions to, produce, edit, and distribute email reminders, target mailings, and newsletters.
- Ensure the placement of new photographs, the development of new topics, and/or the presentation of new ideas on the bulletin boards.
- Develop and maintain a grief-support program to help clients adjust to the loss of their pets. Oversee the:
  1. Mailing of condolence cards
  2. Distribution of paw-print molds, locks of hair, or similar remembrances
  3. Selection of and donations to pet memorials
  4. Selection of crematory services and pet cemeteries that are honest and reliable
  5. Location of and arrangement for contact with grief counselors for anyone in need of assistance
  6. Immediate notification of clients when pets' ashes are returned

CHAPTER 12

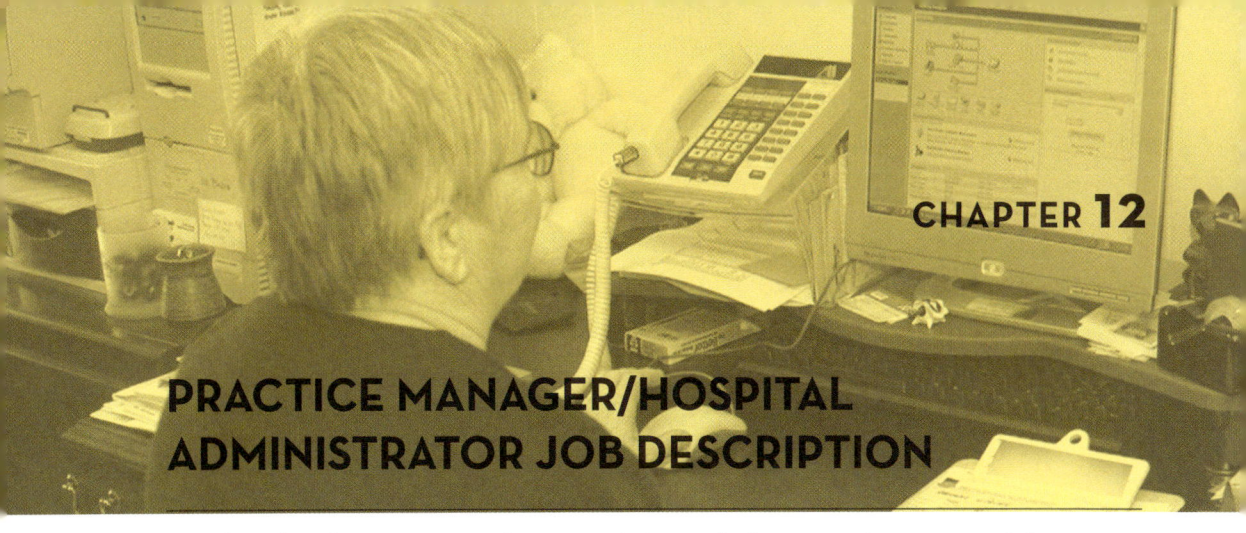

PRACTICE MANAGER/HOSPITAL ADMINISTRATOR JOB DESCRIPTION

Under the direction and supervision of the practice owner(s), practice managers will make many or most of the day-to-day veterinary-practice management decisions. These decisions include financial, budgeting, drug and supplies inventory, marketing, personnel, and facility-management decisions. Because of the complexity of these tasks, successful practice managers should have a bachelor's degree or a minimum of eighteen semester credits in management-related subject material. The most successful practice managers also will have had several years of personnel and financial-management experience in veterinary or related businesses.

People filling this position must possess and exhibit maturity and a high level of integrity; have strong communication, organizational, and financial skills; and be eager and able to train and supervise the support staff. Practice managers or hospital administrators should know how to perform all of the following duties and teach delegable duties to staff members.

General Knowledge and Tasks

General Knowledge
- Be reasonably familiar with breeds and coat colors.
- Follow OSHA standards. Be able to find Material Safety Data Sheets quickly.
- Competently speak and write the English language.
- Competently speak a second language commonly used at the practice.

General Tasks
- Develop and post a personal work schedule so that others will know when you are available. In addition to scheduled hours,

provide home and mobile contact phone numbers, and be available as additional duties and emergency circumstances demand.
- Arrive for work punctually so as to set a good example for staff.
- Maintain a professional appearance while at work, including clean and pressed uniforms or clothes. Change clothes daily as necessary to look professional and avoid carrying odors.
- Smile and maintain an even, friendly demeanor while on the job. Perform job tasks efficiently without rushing.
- Handle stress and pressure with poise and tact.
- Show respect for clients, team members, and animals (alive or deceased) at all times.
- Have the physical strength and ability to lift pets and objects weighing up to 50 pounds without assistance. Assist in lifting patients weighing more than 50 pounds.
- Participate in your performance appraisal.
- Handle communications with staff, doctors, clients, other professionals (CPAs, lawyers), detail reps, and vendors with a professional demeanor.
- Conduct tours of the practice and/or kennel. Before each tour, ensure that the facility is orderly and that staff and patients are prepared for tours.
- Maintain constant vigilance regarding open doorways that could allow pets to escape from the facility.
- Maintain strict confidentiality regarding clients and patients for whom the practice provides veterinary services.
- Be prepared to handle any pet or facility emergency that may arise, including dog or cat fights, choking or strangulating animals, and facility fire or weather-related emergencies. Follow contingency plans.
- Follow established facility closing procedures to ensure the security of patients, staff, data, revenue, inventory, and the building.

Client-Interaction Tasks

- Develop friendly, professional relationships with clients.
- Use clients' and patients' names during conversations.
- Offer financial estimates to clients for services to be performed on patients as directed by doctors. Teach other support staff how to handle this task with confidence and tact.

- Counsel clients on payment options. Enlist doctors or veterinary technicians to answer medical questions or questions requiring medical judgment beyond your expertise.
- Discuss and enforce policies regarding payments, credit, finance fees, and pet health insurance. Assist with CareCredit® applications.
- Review various legal-consent forms with clients, explain them, answer questions, and have clients sign the forms. Check that clients' signatures match the signatures on the records.
- Advise clients of significant changes in policies or services since their last visit.
- Placate and/or compensate clients distressed by long waits, scheduling glitches, and other problems.
- Handle angry or grieving clients with a calm and reassuring manner. Be familiar with the grieving process. Always be sensitive to background chatter or conversations that could exacerbate the anxieties and grief clients experience during euthanasias or deaths of their pets.

Office-Management Tasks

General Office-Management Tasks

- Arrange for waiting-room amenities, such as current magazines, beverages, telephone, and/or television.
- Arrange for the production and distribution of business cards for veterinarians and staff members.
- Understand how to operate all office business machines, including fax machines, copiers, personal digital assistants (PDAs), pagers, and voice-mail or messaging systems.
- Ensure that service reminders and thank-you, welcome, condolence, and birthday cards are all sent in a timely manner.
- Investigate complaints. Resolve complaints in a manner that best supports the practice's mission and philosophy. When appropriate, advise complainants of your findings and the resolutions that address their complaints.
- Evaluate general-business, health, professional-liability, worker's compensation, and/or company-auto insurance policies yearly. Ensure that coverage is current and complete. Periodically seek quotes from alternate companies for comparison.

Phone Tasks

- Know phone functions, including the hold, intercom, transfer, forward, and three-way calling. Know who to call for repairs.
- Arrange for a reliable and cordial answering service, and provide its staff with specific, complete instructions for appropriate greetings, triage, and doctor-on-call contact.
- Establish an appropriate message on the answering machine.

Computer and Internet Tasks

- Program the practice-management software to maintain and search for, store, and print specialized lists from the database, such as:
  1. Patients that are overdue for services and/or refills of pharmaceutical products
  2. Clients with due or overdue balances on their accounts
  3. New patient/client lists
  4. Numbers of new clients per month
  5. Average client transaction or invoice fees (ACTs)
  6. Income production by doctor and groomer
  7. Doctors' average client-transaction or invoice fees (Dr. ACTs)
- Make bookkeeping entries, produce reports, and train others to read data and make entries.
- Draft letters and modify and print forms or letters.
- Assign computer passwords and identification codes to veterinarians and staff members. Ensure codes are properly used so that employees' work can be audited and entries are properly attributed to veterinarians and staff members.
- Access and navigate the Internet to find veterinary websites, order supplies, and access information for clients.
- Design, or contract with a website designer to design, maintain, and/or make improvements to the website using client and staff input. Ensure that the website promotes the practice's mission and goals.
- Assign and maintain email accounts. Check email regularly for clients' and suppliers' questions, requests, and information. Reply to emails or transfer them to appropriate employees.
- Back up computer files at the close of each business day, and ensure the backup is transported and secured at a location off the premises.

Procedure and Policy Tasks

- With the practice owner, veterinarians, and staff, develop core values as well as vision and mission statements for the practice.
- Plan, develop, and coordinate policies and procedures for:
  1. Keeping medical records
  2. Ordering, receiving, stocking, and inventorying drugs and supplies
  3. Dispensing prescription products
  4. Scheduling appointments, surgeries, drop-offs or outpatient procedures, grooming, and boarding
  5. Handling emergency calls during regular business hours and after hours
  6. Scheduling shifts for support and/or doctor staff members, including on-call or emergency schedules
  7. Recording and storing employee time sheets
  8. Creating and implementing effective client reminder systems
- Develop templates for descriptions of procedures and associated fees with the assistance of doctors and/or practice owner(s).
- Develop and use:
  1. Admittance forms
  2. Disclaimers and legal consent forms
  3. New client and patient forms
  4. Inventory control forms
  5. Staff time records
- Develop and maintain an efficient medical record management system. Ensure that files are filed with accuracy and ease, and located quickly. Maintain specific locations or storage bins where active and inactive files are stored while in use.
- Develop, train others in, and follow protocols for handling:
  1. Animal emergencies
  2. Pets that have escaped from the facility
  3. Employees who have been bitten or scratched
  4. Natural disasters, including fires, flooding, hurricanes, and tornados
  5. Internal emergencies, including power losses, fires, dangerous persons
  6. Man-made disasters necessitating rapid exit from the property

Regulatory Tasks

- Be familiar with federal and state regulations regarding pharmacy, controlled-drug, and staffing issues.
- Maintain the physical plant and operations to meet the AAHA Standards of Accreditation or state board minimum standards of practice. Oversee the AAHA accreditation process and follow up on recommended improvements.

Human-Resource Management Tasks

General Human-Resource Tasks

- Promote a positive attitude among staff, and motivate them to carry out the practice's vision and mission.
- Establish a chain of command so that staff members know to whom they should look for initial responses to ethical, medical, business, or personnel problems or concerns.
- Establish work priorities for staff members under your supervision. Maintain an efficient workflow.
- Prepare agendas for, schedule, and lead staff and staff training (including OSHA training) meetings. Ensure that training sessions are useful and productive. Encourage off-site continuing education. Teach other staff members bookkeeping, medical-record-keeping, equipment-maintenance, computer, inventory-management, client-relations, facility-maintenance, and cleaning skills, and about protection against physical and contagious hazards. Keep records of all training meetings.
- Schedule staff to ensure adequate coverage while minimizing downtime and overtime.
- Develop comprehensive personnel policies, development programs, and training programs that encourage applicants to accept job offers, protect and train current employees, and meet financial and quality-assurance goals.
- Develop personnel policies and a personnel policy manual that set standards for:
    1. Hiring
    2. Staff training
    3. Appearance
    4. Performance appraisals

5. Fringe benefits
6. Pay
7. Work schedules
8. Vacations
9. Jury duty
10. Maternity and other leaves of absence
11. Holiday schedules and pay
12. Overtime
13. Continuing education
14. Sick pay
15. Disabilities
16. Complaints regarding discrimination
17. Complaints regarding sexual harassment
18. Conflict resolution
19. Legal notifications
20. Tardiness
21. Personal time
22. Disciplinary action
23. Employment terminations

- Reevaluate and revise policies in the personnel policy manual as needed. (Note: AAHA offers the AAHA Guide to Creating an Employee Handbook, Second Edition to help you achieve this goal.)
- Establish and maintain accurate employee records files in a locked filing cabinet. Protect the confidentiality of such information.

Hiring Tasks

- Develop, use, and maintain job applications for various staff positions.
- Recruit new employees by posting notices, placing classified advertisements, and attending job fairs, and via direct solicitation. Create advertisements for staff positions and determine where to advertise to most effectively fill vacancies.
- Review job applications and resumes. Conduct phone and/or in-person interviews of potential employees. Assess their personalities, intelligence, potential for loyalty and care-giving, enthusiasm, stability, judgment, and technical skills. Check references and, if appropriate, run credit, drug, and background checks.

- When applicants will not be offered employment, inform them within a reasonable time period.
- Offer successful applicants employment and provide details of offers, including start date, initial salary, and benefits. Once the offer has been accepted, complete and submit the new hire paperwork, including:
  1. Payroll information
  2. I-9 verification of work eligibility
  3. W-9 tax withholding
  4. Health-coverage applications
  5. Other fringe benefits forms
- Assign trainers and mentors to new employees. Provide new hires with job descriptions, individualized training schedules, and performance-appraisal forms. Clearly define expectations.

Performance-Appraisal and Termination Tasks

- Regularly evaluate the job performance of staff members. Develop and follow guidelines and appraisal forms to review and evaluate employees' performances. Teach managers to contribute to and conduct evaluations for employees. Teach employees to productively and actively participate in their reviews.
- Participate in the reviews of associate veterinarians. Contribute to the discussion of their client skills, staff interactions, work ethic, and production levels. Ensure that the medical and surgical skills of associate veterinarians are adequate.
- Initiate disciplinary actions against employees. Provide verbal or written warnings for inappropriate work-related behaviors, and clearly state consequences for continued problems. Place employees on probation or suspension for serious or chronic work-related offenses. Document actions.
- Terminate the employment of employees when justified. Conduct exit interviews and, as much as possible, use the information to improve your performance and that of other personnel. Retrieve keys and all property that belongs to the practice. Advise employees of COBRA options, severance pay, and ongoing benefits as appropriate. Document the circumstances of terminations and exit conversations.

Pay and Benefits Tasks

- Set pay levels for each position. Establish clear differentiating skill sets for different pay levels.
- Develop, implement, and manage incentive programs that bond employees to the practice, encourage superior work performance, and keep costs within the budget allocated for staff expenses. Collect and evaluate data from various incentive bonus programs. Distribute bonuses in a timely fashion.
- Determine each doctor's income production, calculate production-based pay, and ensure the distribution of reconciled compensation for doctors at the appropriate monthly or quarterly time intervals.
- Track each doctor's emergency calls, calculate emergency pay, and distribute pay to doctors.
- Oversee payroll. Process time records. Adjust records and pay to account for time used for continuing education, vacation, illness, maternity/paternity leave, personal time, and/or disability. Ensure timely delivery, or automatic deposit, of employee paychecks.
- Evaluate potential fringe benefits programs, and, with the practice owner(s), determine which benefits to offer employees. Consider the benefits and costs of medical and dental health coverage, IRS-qualified profit-sharing and retirement programs, disability insurance, pet health insurance, and continuing education.
- Administer employee benefits. Ensure that employees are aware of the benefits available to them. Enroll new employees in the benefits programs. Complete and submit the required benefits paperwork. Serve as liaison between employees and benefits companies when the needs arise. Deduct established copayments from employees' pay.

Facility and Equipment Tasks

- Ensure regulatory compliance with OSHA, DEA, the State Labor Code, and the state's board of veterinary medicine. Post required agency forms, records, and reports. Administer an OSHA plan or assign and train an OSHA officer.

- Maintain a file of equipment, instruments, furnishings, and product purchase receipts; instruction booklets; and warranties to ensure easy access.
- Maintain a list of contractors, vendors, and service people for repairs, maintenance work, and emergencies.
- Price, evaluate, and purchase equipment service or maintenance agreements.
- Understand the practice-management software. Serve as a resource to staff for training and for resolving computer problems. Contact customer support if needed.
- Maintain and, with the approval of the practice owner(s), update computer hardware and software to maximize the efficiency of the business' computer system. Train staff on upgrades, or arrange for training to ensure a smooth transition.
- Select and purchase office and medical equipment using input from veterinarians and staff.
- Select and purchase reference books for the library using input from veterinarians and owner(s).
- Select, arrange for installation of, and/or maintain the security system. Establish procedures for its use and train staff members accordingly.
- Routinely inspect the facility and ensure the continuous upkeep and maintenance of the buildings, furnishings, and grounds. Contract with landscaping and maintenance firms to provide repairs or maintenance as needed. Assign basic landscaping, mowing, and repair tasks to appropriate staff members or outside vendors.

Financial-Management Tasks

- Protect the business from economic losses due to theft, embezzlement, and negligence by developing internal controls to monitor client payments, bank deposits, and accounts receivable. Maintain tight inventory controls. Carry insurance to protect against theft and embezzlement.
- Prepare monthly and yearly financial and business reports: cash-flow analyses, income statements, balance sheets, and budgets.
- Establish policies regarding client credit, payment schedules, held checks, and the assessment of finance fees. Establish and/or

maintain a credit application and management system for client accounts.

- With input from the practice's owner(s), evaluate and adjust fees at no less than six-month intervals. Refer to AAHA's The Veterinary Fee Reference for guidance. Determine a formula for pharmacy and drug markups. Ensure that fees reflect the owners' goals, the practice's mission, and the practice's target market.
- Maintain accurate records of all revenues, expenses, disbursements, and loans.
- Develop spreadsheets for budgets, cash-flow analyses, schedules, and analyses of potential capital investments.
- Develop and manage a system to track and recover accounts receivable. While following appropriate fair-debt collection laws, complete timely written or oral communications with clients who have overdue accounts, or assign and train another staff person to do this.
- Track accounts payable or supervise the bookkeeper's activities to pay bills in a timely fashion, take advantage of time-sensitive discounts, and avoid late fees, disruption in service, or deterioration of relationships with vendors. Handle reimbursements to staff for travel, continuing education, and other approved miscellaneous expenses.
- Maintain a preset amount of petty cash to use for minor daily cash needs. Track petty cash expenditures, and reconcile this account no less than once monthly.
- Ensure that credit card receipts match statements of credit card income and that credit card debits are only for legitimate client refunds. Confirm that cash and check totals match the receipts recorded as paid by cash and check, respectively. Investigate and resolve discrepancies. Inform owner(s) and CPAs of discrepancies immediately, and confer with them to solve discrepancies.
- Send monthly invoices containing accurately updated finance charges. Properly record payments received. Select a collection agency or attorney to handle accounts that are more than ninety days delinquent, and establish a system to transfer such accounts to these parties.
- Prepare checks for signatures by the owner(s).
- Review and reconcile financial reports, ledgers, and budgets. Reconcile day sheets and income reports daily.

- Develop and maintain an effective relationship with the practice's banker.
- Correspond with and learn from the CPA. Provide the CPA with essential financial records. Respond to inquiries and provide additional information when requested.
- Develop and participate in programs that further the fiscal planning process, including its cash-flow needs, debt repayment, and choices or decisions relative to capital investments.
- Use historical information to forecast future revenues and expenses and develop the practice's and the departmental budgets. Follow budgets when making purchasing and staffing decisions.
- Prepare and implement one-, five-, and ten-year business plans that develop the practice's vision and mission through staff development, facility repairs or expansions, and capital investments.
- Oversee each day's cash receipts and deposits. Establish policies that preclude the same staff member from filling out the deposit slips and making the bank deposits.
- Check credit card company statements to ensure that all credits and debits are accurately recorded in the practice's account.
- Track payable taxes. With the assistance of the CPA, complete and file accurate monthly, quarterly, and annual tax reports.
- Audit employees' work and the practice's procedures. Ensure that procedures are properly followed and that they are effective.

Inventory-Management Tasks

- Oversee and maintain inventory.
- Develop and/or implement an inventory-control system that minimizes theft.
- Develop minimum drug and hospital supply values and reorder points. Train staff to properly use the inventory system, and monitor it for correct use.
- Establish and/or maintain a computerized tracking system for accurately inventorying products and supplies.

Marketing Tasks

- Build friendly, professional relationships with clients, colleagues, detail reps, vendors, and local resources such as animal shelters, city officials, and police.
- Analyze the demographics and psychographics of clientele and potential consumers to properly position the practice and develop marketing materials, including a logo, coordinated stationery, brochures, newsletters, and advertisements.
- Develop programs and marketing materials that enhance clients' experiences, retain clients, and grow visibility within the community.
- Develop, plan, and implement special projects, including open houses, pet fairs, pet-week promotions, and school tours and visits.
- Establish and maintain signs that promote visibility, enhance the practice's appearance, and notify clients of important policies.
- Develop, seek contributions to, produce, edit, and distribute email reminders, direct mail, and newsletters, brochures, and handouts. Periodically evaluate publications for accuracy and contemporary nature of the data; update them as necessary.
- Ensure the placement of new photographs, the development of new topics, and/or the presentation of new ideas on the bulletin boards.
- Develop and maintain a grief-support program to help clients adjust to the loss of their pets. Oversee the:
  1. Mailing of condolence cards
  2. Distribution of paw-print molds, locks of hair, or similar remembrances
  3. Selection of donations to pet memorials
  4. Selection of urns, crematory services, and pet cemeteries that are honest and reliable
  5. Location of and arrangement for contact with grief counselors for anyone in need.
  6. Immediate notification of clients when pets' ashes are returned

RESOURCES

"The ADA Guide to Preparing Job Descriptions." The University of Delaware. www.udel.edu/ADA/hiring.html.

Garner, Candy, Tom Catanzaro, DVM, Jim Shirey, DVM, et al. *AAHA Guide to Creating an Employee Handbook*, Second Edition. AAHA Press, 1999.

Gendron, Karen, DVM. *A Practical Guide to Performance Appraisals.* AAHA Press, 2002.

The Guide to Writing Job Descriptions. College and Professional Association for Human Resources, 1992. www.cupahr.org/hrpubs/details/guideada.htm.

Handling Basic Employment Discrimination Cases and/or To Accommodate or Not To Accommodate: What's Reasonable, What's Substantial and Other ADA Questions. The Association of the Bar of the City of New York. 212/382-6663; www.abcny.org.

Hill's Veterinary Nutritional Advocate Training. Enables support-staff members to receive nutrition counseling and a certificate. www.hillspet.com.

LifeLearn Staff Training Series. Available through AAHA Press.

Protecting Pets. Protecting People. The Zoonotic Educational Study Guide and Protecting Your Patients, Protecting Your Practice: Important Issues for 2004. us.merial.com.

Templates for *Estimates by Diagnosis*. Veterinary Management Consultation, Inc. 303/674-8169.

The Veterinary Fee Reference, Fourth Edition. AAHA Press, 2005.

VPI eUniversity staff training information regarding pet health insurance. vets.petinsurance.com.

Wilson, James, DVM, JD, and Charlotte Lacroix. *Legal Consent Forms for Veterinary Practices*. Priority Press, 2001. Available through AAHA Press.

Wilson, James, DVM, JD, and C. McConnell, DVM, MBA. *Veterinary Receptionist's Training Manual*. Priority Press, 1998. Available through AAHA Press.